A Personal Touch On...™ Celiac Disease

Written by:
People Touched By Celiac
Sharing Stories To Help You

edited by:
Peter R. Berlin
Jerry Stone

A Personal Touch Publishing, LLC.
Los Angeles, California

APT Publishing

Printed in the United States of America

ISBN 0-9748566-0-6

Library of Congress Control Number: 2004090347

Publisher: A Personal Touch Publishing, LLC.
　　　　　1335 La Brea Avenue #2
　　　　　Los Angeles, California 90028
　　　　　www.apersonaltouchon.com

Cover Design by Gary Solomon/gsdstudio.com

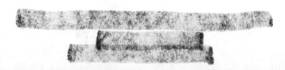

To Tyler McKinley, age seven, whose courage and perseverance was the inspiration for this book.

To all those who have celiac disease, diagnosed or undiagnosed, who live through this everyday. We encourage you to pave the path for others.

What lies behind us and what lies before us are tiny matters compared to what lies within us.

- Oliver Wendell Holmes

Table Of Contents

1. Finding Out What's Wrong
I Thought M.D. Meant "Medical Doctor," Not "Missed Diagnosis"

2. Celiac: An Inherited Disease
Why Couldn't You Just Leave Me The House?

3. My New Life
Wheat No More, My Baby

4. Living With Celiac
Showing Real Intestinal Fortitude

5. My Child Has Celiac
Kids Contract The Darndest Things

6. Making It Easier For Our Children
No Kidding

7. Being A Teen With Celiac
As If Acne Wasn't Bad Enough

8. Senior Celiacs
Ain't No Stopping Me Now

9. Success With Celiac
You Don't Have To Be A Gluten For Punishment

10. Travel Tales
Don't Forget To Pack Your Gluten-Free Food

11. Recipes For Success
Now You're Cooking

12.Tips, Tricks And Smiles
Some Simple Celiac Solutions

Acknowledgements

by Peter R. Berlin

For the past 25 plus years, I have been in the television industry where I produced and wrote for many game and talk shows. One of the benefits of that career is knowing a lot of trivia, including how many newborn baby opossums can fit in a teaspoon (18), and the fact that Reno is farther west than Los Angeles. Having mastered this talent (I am a real threat in any Trivial Pursuit game I enter) I have moved into the world of book publishing with my longtime friend, Jerry Stone. This is the first in what we hope will be many books in which people will be able to help others by sharing their experiences.

I t's hard to imagine that last fall, "A Personal Touch On...™," was just an idea. A series of books designed to inform, inspire, encourage, and give hope to the reader, written solely by people willing to share their first hand experiences. The response was tremendous and now several months later, the first in this exciting series is about to be published. This accomplishment is due to the efforts and help of a lot of people and to the accessibility provided by the Internet. So the first acknowledgement goes to the host of on-line search engines and forums that allowed us to spread the word and get in touch with those "out there" who contributed to this project. In the same way the Internet helped us compile the book, it is an incredible source of information for those with celiac disease. Here are a few of the helpful sites we visited: the Celiac Listserv at www.enabling.org/ia/celiac, Delphi forum at www.delphi.com, and celiac.com. The message boards on these sites are invaluable sources of information with many wonderful people sharing their experiences to help others. I highly recommend them to everybody looking for information or "someone to talk to."

In order to be able to obtain the submissions for this book we needed a Web site. Thank you, Bradley Stone, for all your hard work and incredible skill in putting up a site in a timely manner that was user friendly.

The design of the Web site and cover of the book is due to the wonderful talent of Gary Solomon of gsdstudio.com. Gary's design which melds the medical with the personal wonderfully conveys the spirit of the book.

Thanks to Jim Bontempo for your work in the editing process and to Howie Kuperberg for your clever thoughts.

Thanks to Beverly Berlin and Donna Stone for your love, support, and hard work.

Several individuals in the celiac community were extremely helpful and supportive in getting the word out about our project. Special thanks to Melonie Katz, who runs a terrific on-line support group at yahoo.com. Melonie, you were there at the beginning offering support, advice, and help by opening the door to others in the celiac community. Your on-line group mirrors the philosophy of the book by taking a positive attitude to celiac disease and the gluten-free lifestyle. For readers out there who would like information about joining this group you can e-mail Melonie at SillyYaks-subscribe@yahoogroups.com. I would like to also thank Melonie for contributing several pieces including the introduction "What Is Celiac Disease?"

We found an incredible amount of information on-line at The Sprue-Nik Press published by the Tri-County Celiac Sprue Support Group, serving southeastern Michigan. They put out a comprehensive newsletter and have a wonderful archive of past editions which can be reached through the Celiac Listserv. Several of the pieces in this book were submitted by people whose work appeared on-line in Sprue-Nik's newsletter. Thank you, to those people who updated and submitted their pieces to us.

Thanks to Sue Goldstein and Leslie Elsner, who served as co-editors of the Westchester Celiac Sprue Support Group newsletter, for their help in putting us in contact with several of the people whose pieces appear in this book.

Thanks to Clan Thompson at www.clanthompson.com for putting a piece about our efforts in your newsletter. Numerous people responded to your posting and sent us their stories.

Thank you to Sue Clayton of the Gluten-Free Group of Arizona, Lucy Shriver of The Gluten-Free Kitchen and LynnRae Ries at www.whatnowheat.com for spreading the word to your group's members.

Thanks to Mary Guerriero, of Tri-County Celiac Sprue Support Group and Marge Johannemann, of Greater Louisville Celiac Sprue Support Group, for not only contributing pieces, but for putting us in contact with several other members of the celiac community.

Thanks to Anne Barfield, of the San Antonio Celiac

Sprue Support Group, William Lucas, of the South Jersey Celiac Support Group, and Beverly Chevalier, co-founder of the greater New Haven Support Group, for helping us make contact with several contributors.

Thanks to all who took the time and effort to write and submit pieces for publication. It is your caring and willingness to share that will inspire, encourage, give hope to, and inform those who have celiac disease and those who may not yet know they have it. Your efforts will go a long way to help many others.

And last but not least, a very special thanks to Danna Korn for your input, and for writing the foreword to this book. Your tireless work and selfless dedication to helping others with celiac is only exceeded by your positive attitude and approach to the work.

One last note. If I've learned one thing in the last few months it is there are many wonderful and generous people out there willing to help others by giving of their time and information. There are many celiac support groups all over the country with people ready and willing to share their experiences. If you have celiac disease or gluten intolerance; join a group, get involved. Learn from people who have experienced what you are going through and then help those who come after you. The benefits to you and others will be tremendous.

Foreword

by Danna Korn

I've been involved in the celiac world since 1991, when my then-toddler son, Tyler, was diagnosed. At that time, there were very few resources, no support groups for kids on the gluten-free diet, and no internet. We felt truly on an island. As I learned to deal with it -- not dwell on it (my mantra) -- I felt compelled to reach out and help others. I started R.O.C.K. (Raising Our Celiac Kids), wrote two books, and speak around the country on living -- and loving -- the gluten-free lifestyle. Today, we realize that Tyler's diagnosis has actually been a huge blessing in our lives. How privileged we are to be able to help others realize that this can be a blessing in their lives, too.

The very basis of this book is that it is written by people whose lives have been touched by celiac disease for people with celiac disease, providing support and inspiration from people who have actually "been there, done that." The stories are written from the heart and will help you realize you're not alone in your struggles. After reading these pieces you will never have to say, "nobody knows what I'm going through." We can go to the Internet or to our doctors for facts, but this book gives you more. It gives you the ability to learn from the experiences of others. This book touches on many different aspects of celiac disease, from many different points of view, by taking a warm, human, non-clinical approach. The range of stories and contributors is impressive. From a six-year-old girl, who tells about her first gluten-free Halloween, to a senior citizen, who tells of how she finally got a diagnosis at the age of 67, after years of suffering with an "unknown" ailment.

My personal touch on celiac disease is from the perspective of a parent of a celiac child, and the myriad of emotions that we parents experience knowing our children will be gluten-free for the rest of their lives.

My "PollyDanna" nature urges me to skip to the current chapter in our lives, when we have learned to live – and love – this gluten-free lifestyle, and to appreciate the fact that our son was diagnosed, when we know most people with celiac disease will never hold the key to better health, as we do. But to convince you we truly do understand the challenges, I'm compelled to share the difficulties we faced, albeit in a highly abbreviated form, in order to reach the point where we are today: thankful for our gluten-freedom (I never was good at saving the punch line till the end).

As a toddler, our son was sick. It seemed to me he was dying, as his belly grew distended and his personality transformed from a happy, energetic nine-month-old to a listless, lethargic, irritable 18-month-old. Yet not one, not two, but three pediatricians sent us away – fired us, in fact – and said there was nothing wrong with our child. They told us to load him up on cookies, crackers, breads – anything to "plug" him up, as the diarrhea was nearly unmanageable. Little did I know, I was poisoning him with every bite.

After a long nine months, four pediatricians, a pediatric

gastroenterologist, and dozens of hospital tests later, Tyler was diagnosed with celiac disease. It was 1991, and celiac disease was still thought to be a rare, pediatric condition. We know today, of course, that it is neither. We were sent forth to live our lives without gluten, and instructed to load up on Rice Krispies and Corn Flakes (both of which we quickly found out contained gluten). Yes, we were truly, or at least we felt, on an island.

Those of us who once felt on an island better hope it's a big one, because we now know that celiac disease is the most common genetic disease of mankind. Thankfully, today we have good resources, great-tasting and more readily available gluten-free products, and excellent support organizations.

This book, from the perspective of people who have been touched by celiac disease reaches out to inspire and support others with celiac disease. It offers a profound and insightful look at the unique challenges we face, and how others have overcome those challenges to embrace this lifestyle with the realization that it is truly the key to better health.

Whether you're newly diagnosed, searching for guidance and assurance that everything will, in fact, be okay, or an old pro, easily working your way through complex labels and lengthy safe/forbidden ingredients lists, this book will provide inspiration and encouragement from those who have truly "been there, done that."

Danna is the author of "Wheat-Free, Worry-Free: The Art of Happy, Healthy, Gluten-Free Living" and "Kids With Celiac Disease: A Family Guide To Raising Happy, Healthy, Gluten-Free Children." Her new Web site GlutenFreedom.net is dedicated to help inform and educate people who are on, or are considering the wheat-free/gluten-free diet.

What Is Celiac Disease?
by Melonie Katz

I'm the mom of a two-and-a-half-year-old celiac toddler who has been gluten-free since she was diagnosed at 19 months. Her distended tummy and a dozen diarrhea diapers a day led me to research information on the Internet. I suspected celiac disease almost immediately, but it took four long months of visits with twenty four different healthcare professionals before she was actually diagnosed. Raising a gluten-free child does have its challenges, but we've embraced the challenge with welcome arms. I have an on-line support group and extend an invitation for others to join by sending me an e-mail at SillyYaks-subscribe@yahoogroups.com.

Celiac disease is condition that affects nearly 1 in every 133 Americans. There are the people who know they have celiac disease because they have received a medical diagnosis, and then there are even more people who have yet to be diagnosed. Celiac disease is often not diagnosed due to lack of awareness and education. Diagnosis can also be difficult because often times the symptoms of celiac disease are not always the typical "GI" sorts of problems. Someone can even be celiac without showing obvious symptoms. There have been estimates that two million undiagnosed celiacs are in the United States alone. Could you be one of them?

So, what is celiac disease? It is a genetic autoimmune disorder that presents itself with a variety of symptoms or no symptoms at all. Sometimes the symptoms can include, but are not limited to: diarrhea, constipation, vomiting, headaches, food intolerances, malnutrition, weight loss or weight gain, and the list really continues. Unfortunately, many people show no real symptoms at all, or their symptoms have led to a misdiagnosis. Generally, someone lives with celiac disease for many years before getting the bittersweet diagnosis.

A few conditions must be present for someone to have celiac disease. First, you must be genetically predisposed to having it. In other words, you must have one of the two genes that have been linked to celiac disease. Secondly, you must be eating a diet that contains gluten. And lastly, there must be what is called an "environmental trigger" that causes celiac disease to present itself. An environmental trigger is a stressor on the body such as a virus, major illness, pregnancy, etc. However, not everyone who is genetically predisposed for celiac disease will develop it.

If you have celiac disease, your body recognizes gluten as a toxin. Toxins are essentially poisons to your body. Gluten wreaks havoc on a celiac's body. First and foremost, gluten causes the villi, which line the intestinal wall, to become flattened and lose the ability to absorb nutrients from foods. Therefore, if you have celiac disease you must avoid all gluten (wheat, rye, barley, and their derivatives). It means you must maintain a gluten-free lifestyle, for life. It is a HEALTHY lifestyle and it is a wonderful "prescription for life." There are no surgeries, no lifelong dependency on medications, and no real "side effects."

Over time, your body can make a full recovery if you maintain a gluten-free diet.

Living with celiac disease means changing your lifestyle, modifying your diet, being willing to accept change and persevere. It means becoming an expert at reading ingredient labels, calling food manufacturers to clarify food sources, asking questions at restaurants, choosing not to eat foods at social events, bringing healthy gluten-free foods to food related functions, and taking extra time for planning and preparation of gluten-free meals. It also means knowing more about yourself and your diet than the average person. Is that so bad? To know the ingredients of what you use to fuel your body? Absolutely not!

It means finding others, sharing stories, joining and forming support groups. It means you have already learned a lot, just by reading "A Personal Touch on...Celiac Disease." The shared experiences in this book will tell you even more about celiac disease and what it is like to live with it.

Finding Out What's Wrong

I Thought M.D. Meant "Medical Doctor," Not "Missed Diagnosis"

> *My villi they are compromised,*
> *It took dozens of doctors to surmise.*
> *Now they know what is wrong,*
> *With my diet I'm strong.*
> *My life and my outlook revived.*

Long Road To Diagnosis
by Tina Ackerman

Hi, I'm Tina Ackerman, a 25-year-old, living in Goffstown, New Hampshire. I was finally diagnosed with Celiac Sprue in May 2003. My favorite grocery store to shop at is Trader Joe's. They have a gluten-free spicy jalapeno chicken sausage that simply ROCKS!

During my senior year of college, I had to work full time to support myself. My parents are not wealthy so they were only able to help me with love and support, not financially.

By the end of October, I was very tired and not feeling up to par. My co-workers suggested I go to the emergency room to be evaluated since I had no physician. I figured I caught a virus or was just run down since I was in school and working so much. The ER ran all kinds of tests including blood work, a mono screen, a strep test, a complete blood count, and a metabolic panel. Everything came back normal. They said I had a virus that caused gastroenteritis. This is how they explained the abdominal pain and diarrhea.

I returned to work and school, just trying to survive each day. Weeks passed and I did not feel any better. I completely stopped eating because it was hard to keep food down. When

I wasn't vomiting, I had horribly painful abdominal cramping and persistent diarrhea. My weight went from 110 to 90 pounds. Since my condition wasn't improving, I went to the doctor at the local Family Health Center. The nurse practitioner I saw was worried I had cholecystitis (inflammation of the gallbladder). She ordered an ultrasound and made an appointment for me with a surgeon. They cancelled the appointment when the results of the ultrasound came back normal.

I was extremely frustrated. While I didn't want something to be wrong, I wanted to find out what was causing my problems so I could feel better. I was so tired and dehydrated I would pass out if I stood up quickly. I went back to the nurse practitioner a few days later and this time they admitted my 87 pound emaciated body into the hospital. They ran more tests and drew lots of blood. The test results were all negative. They decided I had irritable bowel syndrome (IBS) and referred me to a gastroenterologist. The doctor placed me on Levsin for the abdominal cramping. This helped but I began to have side effects from the medication. I had trouble urinating and became extremely sensitive to light. I stopped taking the medication.

Since she couldn't find anything physically wrong with me, she concluded I must be depressed, anxious, and making myself sick.

The doctor then told me to go on a BRAT (Banana, Rice, Applesauce, and Toast) diet. This bland diet was supposed to help my stomach get used to digesting food again.

My health was so bad I took a leave of absence from school and work and moved back with my parents for a month to recover. I slowly began to feel better.

A few months later I began to date my future husband, Tom. I was often embarrassed when we first started dating. We would be out shopping or at a movie and we would have to stop what we were doing and go home because of my "IBS". When the diarrhea came it would be horrible, painful, and physically draining. Thankfully Tom took it all in stride. It did not bother him that I was gassy, bloated, and miserable a lot of the time. It was very emotionally draining for me. I was becoming very self-conscious and had trouble using public restrooms. Being chronically sick took a toll on my self-esteem. I was extremely frustrated with the fact I would be sick for the rest of my life. Slowly I began to gain weight and grew accustomed to all my gastrointestinal distress.

I found myself a new primary care physician and made an appointment for a physical. At the physical I mentioned all my intestinal problems. The doctor ran some tests and like before they all came back negative. Since she couldn't find anything physically wrong with me, she concluded I must be depressed, anxious, and making myself sick.

I was devastated and cried for days. If I wasn't depressed before, I was now. I couldn't imagine why I hated myself so much that I would make myself so sick. I started going to therapy to discover the root of this self-hatred that was making me so ill. The therapist placed me on medications. I went through Paxil, BuSpar, Amitriptyline, Celexa, Ativan, Ambien, Effexor, Klonopin, Prozac, and then Serzone in the course of three years. When one medication didn't work they just put me on another. I stopped taking medication shortly after I started Serzone because I had an allergic reaction. I finally said enough. No more medications.

Four-and-a-half years after my first hospitalization my weight had ballooned to 140 pounds. I was getting married to the love of my life, Tom, and we planned our wedding at the Polynesian Resort at Walt Disney World. Our wedding was perfect, right down to the best cake I had ever tasted and the mouse ears on our heads. We spent five days at Disney World and then took a four day cruise to the Bahamas. We ate and drank like kings. Tom gained 15 pounds in two weeks. I imbibed more than I ever had before. Unfortunately my stomach and intestines were not as happy as my heart and soul. I just felt like hell.

Three weeks after we came back from Florida we went to Baltimore where I attended a John's Hopkins conference for work. Tom came with me even though he had the flu. Wednesday, our first night in Baltimore, we went to the Cheesecake Factory for dinner. I thought I caught Tom's flu because I was nauseous and had abdominal cramping. For dinner I ordered a turkey sandwich of which I only had a few bites. The dessert was the real reason we went to the Cheesecake Factory. I ordered Chocolate Peanut Butter Cheesecake and was only able to eat a quarter of the piece. Tom realized I was not feeling well at this point. I would never pass up a piece of cheesecake. I had been looking forward to eating there for months. By Sunday, I could barely keep any food down. The plane flight home was miserable because I felt so ill. Tom's flu hadn't lasted this long and he already felt normal.

The next day at work was very busy and we had sandwiches delivered for lunch. After eating a quarter of a sandwich, I was sick to my stomach. My abdominal pain was all on the right side. What if I have appendicitis?

I left work and went to the emergency room because my doctor's office could not fit me in. I had a negative CT scan but my white blood cell count was elevated and I was severely dehydrated. So they admitted me into the hospital for three days. The diagnosis came back as "acute exacerbation" of irritable bowel syndrome. My primary care physician told me it was probably due to too much stress in my life. I should change my diet and eat more fiber. She suggested introducing whole wheat products.

I now know I have to be my own advocate and not believe everything a doctor has to say.

Even after being discharged from the hospital I still couldn't eat and lost 10 pounds in two weeks. I spent more time in the emergency room for pain and nausea control and finally begged my doctor to refer me to a gastroenterologist after losing 20 pounds. I was able to make an appointment but had to wait a month.

When I finally had my appointment, the doctor drew some lab work that included a transglutaminase titer (Ttg) for celiac disease. A week later the gastroenterologist called me at work and told me my Ttg was 39. He felt at that level I didn't need a small bowel biopsy to confirm the diagnosis of celiac disease unless I wanted one. I didn't want one.

I had read up on celiac disease so I knew what it was. I would have to be gluten-free for the rest of my life and I would be happy to do that if it made me feel better.

I was happy, angry, and scared all at once. Happy I finally

knew the reason I had been so sick for half my life, angry at my doctors, who misdiagnosed me for so long and who blamed me for being sick, and scared I would never enjoy food again. I love pasta, pizza, and convenience foods and wasn't quite sure how I'd live without them.

I had a follow-up appointment with my primary care physician, who in my opinion, is incompetent and not very empathetic. When I requested a Dexa Scan to measure my bone density she told me I didn't need it. I asked my gastroenterologist at my next appointment if I should have the scan and he agreed I should. The results came back as severely osteopenic. This reinforced the feelings I had about my primary care physician. I now take daily calcium in the form of gluten-free VIACTIV chews. This is so important especially since I was extremely lactose intolerant for the first three months after being diagnosed. Lactose intolerance is very common when the small bowel is healing from all the damage the uncontrolled celiac disease created.

It has been six months since my diagnosis. I am starting to get over my anger about being misdiagnosed and I'm more at ease with myself now. I don't stay up at night thinking about my celiac disease anymore. I now know I have to be my own advocate and not believe everything a doctor has to say. I am the only one who knows when I am sick.

I am learning that being gluten-free isn't the end of your life, it is the beginning. It just takes extra time to plan your meals.

I have traveled to Germany since my diagnosis and had a wonderful experience. I didn't starve while there and actually ate very well. I refuse to get a salad with no dressing every time I go out to eat. You can usually get whatever you want if you explain how it needs to be prepared. This of course applies to real restaurants with chefs, not chain restaurants.

Just read and learn as much as you can. Every celiac needs to learn as much as they can about their condition. Nobody can do it for you. There are wonderful Web sites and books out there that are a tremendous help.

I also try to educate as many people as I can without being annoying. You'll be surprised how many people want to understand this illness. I feel the more we educate people about celiac disease the easier it will be for the afflicted people who are not yet diagnosed.

Celiac Colored Glasses
by Leah Edelstein

*I have an M.S. in speech-language pathology. Currently, I'm
the Co-Chairperson of the Southern New Jersey Chapter of Celiac
Sprue Association/ USA, Inc. My 21-year-old daughter is a senior
at Yale University. My husband and I celebrated our 25th wedding
anniversary in December 2003.*

My friend Fran tells me I see the world through "Celiac Colored Glasses." Allow me to backtrack. I was diagnosed with celiac disease 21 years ago. This was after 10 years of intermittently feeling ill to various degrees. After an emergency hospitalization at age 19 (I had extreme abdominal cramps) I was diagnosed with colitis. Fast forward nine years to less than two months after my daughter was born. I began to have the "classic" symptoms of celiac disease: diarrhea, weight loss, weakness, etc. The doctor dismissed my concerns about my fatigue. He told me my baby was getting heavier to carry (in my arms) and that was why I was feeling so tired. He was clueless. When I began having numbness I asked him to refer me to a neurologist. He did.

I credit that neurologist with saving my life. At first he thought I was malingering (faking illness) but then he did a simple reflexive type test which proved my calcium levels were extremely low. I heard him call my family physician and practically yell at him.

Not too long after, I woke up very early one morning with a complete sensation something was utterly wrong with me. I left my infant daughter with my mom and had my husband drive me to a nearby hospital emergency room. I saw no one in charge and waited patiently. Suddenly someone who seemed

The hospital staff didn't make things less confusing for me. They kept giving me bread with my meals.

to be having a heart attack was rushed through the office door and got attention. I obviously wasn't a top priority. I was finally let in a room and while waiting for a resident my body began to "cramp up." My hands were unable to get out of a fist position. The pain I felt was so much worse than the pain I felt with my then recent experience of natural childbirth. I actually begged my husband to kill me.

When I finally saw a resident I told him about my calcium levels and he began administering calcium through an IV. After my blood work was done it was discovered I needed more than just calcium. I was now a top priority.

Eventually, my body began to feel better. I was attached to a cardiac monitor. Later I learned from a too truthful doctor I was in real danger of going into cardiac arrest. He said it was a miracle I was alive (my electrolyte levels were so low). I found out he wasn't exaggerating when a second doctor repeated the same thing to me a few days later.

Being naive, I thought once I was stabilized I could be discharged. No such luck. I spent 15 days in the hospital and had a different diagnosis almost each day. Finally the results of my small intestinal biopsy returned positive and I was told I had celiac disease. I actually laughed. I told my doctor it was the funniest diagnosis yet! I found it incredible having eaten wheat, rye, oats, and barley for the 28 years of my life that I now had a problem with those grains.

The hospital staff didn't make things less confusing for me. They kept giving me bread with my meals. And being newly diagnosed, with little information about the diet, I ate it. I kept telling myself it must be "special bread," the staff must know what they're doing! I've grown to learn never take anything for granted.

One thing the difficult ordeal of getting a celiac diagnosis has taught me is to suspect celiac in others. The symptoms are so varied and some people don't even have symptoms. According to one respectable source, 97% of celiacs still go undiagnosed. I "see" celiac among many people whom I meet. That's why Fran tells me I see the world through "Celiac Colored Glasses." And what's more, I've influenced her to do the same! ✍

You Have A Disease...
Good Luck!

by Alison St. Sure

*I was diagnosed in December 2002 at the age of 32. I live an
active lifestyle in San Francisco that includes sports, travel, and even
dining out.*

My mom found out I had celiac disease on the
Internet! I had been undergoing blood tests,
including a bone marrow test, to find out why
I was so anemic. At least five doctors had mentioned anemia
over the previous 10 years but had never treated it seriously. I
also experienced stomach trouble for a long time however it
never occurred to me this was not normal. When I told my
mother about my various health problems, she began a search
on the Web and found celiac disease.

After a blood test (which I had to ask for) and a
subsequent biopsy which came back positive, I met with the
gastroenterologist who performed the biopsy. I asked, "So,
how many cases of celiac disease have you diagnosed?" I'm
not sure what number I expected to hear, somewhere around
25? 100? "You're the first!" he replied, as though I had won

some kind of lottery! I had walked into the doctor's office that day thinking what I had was common, but there I stood, shocked and wondering if I was a freak.

I had come prepared with 100 pages I had printed out from the Internet on celiac disease, excited and ready to discuss it all with the doctor: The hidden forms of gluten, the various symptoms and related diseases associated with it, the possible nutritional deficiencies I might have as a result of the damage. Instead I watched the doctor open a big medical textbook to a page on celiac sprue... He said, "So, it looks like you need to stay away from..." He put on his reading glasses and scanned a page of the book. "Wheat..." he turned the page "...Barley, and Rye." End of sentence. End of diagnosis. End of medical advice. "ARE YOU KIDDING ME?" I shouted. Okay, I only shouted it in my head, but it was loud!

I walked out of the office, realizing I would need to figure this out on my own, and headed for a grocery store to get started on my new diet. I was excited and determined when I went in, but burst into tears as I drove away from the store. I wasn't crying because I couldn't eat a muffin anymore, I was crying for the loss of freedom I suddenly felt. I went through a grieving process and have had ups and downs since. Now, almost a year after going gluten-free, I am thankful for the amazing improvement in my health. I am also thankful to my mom for discovering my condition. It turns out she too has celiac disease and we are both living healthier, happier gluten-free lives!

Two Years Of Testing

by Dimitrios Douros

My son Pablo and I were diagnosed in the Spring of 2000. Since then our family has gotten involved in listservs, groups, meetings, the celiac walks, and activities to raise celiac disease awareness and enact food labeling laws.

I didn't know I had celiac disease. I found out after two years of taking my son to general practitioners and specialists. I needed to find out why, even though he ate everything we put in front of him, he had a bloated belly and had not grown an inch or gained a pound from age two to four!

The gastrointestinal specialist said it was constipation and had us give him laxatives! He developed rectal prolapse from straining so hard during his bowel movements. Rectal prolapse is a rare symptom of celiac disease so the doctor missed the diagnosis and tested him for cystic fibrosis, a fatal disease for which rectal prolapse is more common.

I wigged out! I told my wife: "I am not ready to bury my son!"

While the doctor tested him for cystic fibrosis (sweat test) I took matters into my own hands. I went on the Web, and using rectal prolapse as the search item, I looked for a more palatable diagnosis. One of the links took me to a page describing celiac disease. I read the list of symptoms with tears rolling down my cheeks because not only did it fit my son's problems but I also had each and every symptom.

The cystic fibrosis test was negative and we spent the next three to four weeks trying to convince the gastrointestinal specialist to test for celiac disease. She finally did, probably just to shut us up. And guess what! The test was positive so she wanted a confirming biopsy. Our son was just four at the time and hated needles. So I was in the examining room with four other people holding him still so they could hook up the IV for anesthesia! Then I held his hand while the anesthetic was administered. I felt him and saw him go dead limp. I'll never forget it!

My son's biopsy confirmed celiac disease. He went gluten-free, his bloated belly went away and he's been growing like a weed ever since! A month later I had a blood test. It came back negative. But I KNEW I HAD CELIAC! I went gluten-free and ALL my symptoms disappeared in less than a week!

If I didn't hate needles even more than my son, I might have gone for the biopsy to confirm I have celiac disease despite the fact that my blood test was negative. But I do hate needles, so I will not have a confirmed diagnosis.

Finally, what hurts the most about this experience has been to recount and re-live the pain of our two year search for a diagnosis. It upsets me how we had to expend so much energy to demand 21st century medicine to get a diagnosis rather than settle for folksy-wisdom-simple, it-worked-for-my-neighbor remedies.

Finally A Diagnosis

by Joy Moore

*I am 42 years old, a wife of 18 years and a mother to a nine -
year-old daughter, Amanda. I have worked the past two years as a
Food Service Cafeteria Worker at Amanda's school. Imagine the
challenge I live daily as I cook and serve food to nearly 600 students
each day. Hope this is encouraging to you that a gluten-free diet is
manageable with willpower, determination, and yes, even prayer.*

My name is Joy Moore and I have celiac sprue
disease. I have seen so many doctors, too
numerous to count! It all began back in 1986
when I would complain about, you know, the typical
symptoms: bloating, diarrhea, constipation, nausea, joint
pain, and those nagging women issues.

Let me explain how a diagnosis came about after so many
years. In November 2002, I had eaten some food that had
been sitting out from the Thanksgiving meal (bad idea, don't
do it). By December 5th I had been rushed to the emergency
room thinking I was having a heart attack. The doctors ruled
out my heart. I thanked God! With no answers, I was released
from the hospital. I went to my primary care doctor the very
next day and discovered my white blood count was elevated.

After the first ten-day regiment of antibiotics I returned to the doctor still feeling something was seriously wrong with me. A test had been run and an H.Pylori bacteria infection was the culprit. AHH MY TRIGGER!

More antibiotics AND a referral to a gastroenterologist followed. The endoscopy report came back to my primary care manager (quack, oh, I meant the doctor). He took out a scrap piece of paper and jotted down celiac sprue. He handed it to me and said, "Go look this up on the Internet. I think it has to do with wheat." Needless to say he is no longer my doctor. The gastroenterologist confirmed celiac disease by biopsy and sent me off to see a nutritionist to start me on a gluten-free diet. Unfortunately she had never dealt with a celiac patient either. I guess what I am trying to say is that it is your body, your health and your well-being. Be persistent and get the help you need.

A year has passed and sure I feel better since being on the gluten-free diet, but the damage the disease has caused over the years still lingers on. I still suffer from joint pain, mood swings, and those female issues.

Let me end my story with a word of encouragement: sure some days are hard as I watch my family eat a Papa John's Pizza (I can almost taste it) but I know the bite I don't take means another day of healing and improved health.

May God give you the strength and encouragement that you need each day to stay gluten-free.

God Bless. ✒

Confessions Of An Undiagnosed Celiac

by Jeanne Donnelly

I am the mother of two teenage children (both recently diagnosed with celiac disease). I manage an International Student Exchange program based in New Jersey. My hobbies include writing fiction and painting and I hold a black belt in Karate.

D o I have celiac disease? I believe so. As a matter of fact I made myself very sick trying to prove it. What can I say? I was desperate! I spent the past twenty-five years doing everything the doctors told me and I was getting sicker instead of better. All I concentrated on was eating healthy and doing anything that promised to settle my stomach. Nothing worked. Every doctor I complained to ran a few tests and said I probably had irritable bowel syndrome. Their advice was lose weight and watch what I eat. Easy for them to say.

Since it wasn't the in bed, out of work, desperately ill, kind of sick (yet!), I did my best to manage daily life. For the most part my family understood I had a "sensitive stomach" and learned to live with it, but I knew it was slowly getting worse and I was getting scared. Finally, I came to the point where I would just break down and pray to God, "I don't care what it is, just give me an answer. Any answer!"

When I first explained to doctors that I seemed to be always in the bathroom with severe nausea, stomach cramps, gas, and bloating they said, "Must be something you ate." To which, I'd answer, "Everyday?" and they would just shrug their shoulders. It wasn't like I was dying, losing vast amounts of weight or exhibiting symptoms that would raise the red flag, but I was in pain and embarrassed. I don't think the doctors realized what it took for me to come forward with my complaints. As before, I left the doctor's office without any answers and went on with life, managing it as best I could.

My biggest question was why could I eat something one day and be fine, then eat it a week later and be extremely sick? The medical community answered with "It's IBS."

One minute I could feel fine and the next I would be overcome with cramps. Some days I could barely manage to leave the house. It got so bad I would just not eat as I tried to "shut down" the digestive process.

Doctors kept saying irritable bowel syndrome. Frankly, I didn't think that was much of a diagnosis. I mean, I already knew my bowels were irritated! What causes it? What can I do about it?

I was told again, "everyone gets it." Watch what you eat, avoid junk food, alcohol, etc. Yeah right, I'd been trying that for years and it didn't work. One day I'd eat something and be fine, the next day I'd eat the same thing and get sick. What did that tell me? I'd keep food diaries, take vitamins (even those made me nauseous) and on and on but I wasn't feeling any better.

Finally, I resigned myself to carrying a pack of Imodium in my purse wherever I went. It was so bad that everything I ate caused pain. If I had to do any traveling I would just not eat the day before or the day of trip. Everywhere I went I just resigned myself to not eat. Once I got home and felt safe I would be so hungry I would stuff everything I could find into my mouth. Of course, that would make me sick as a dog.

My biggest question was why could I eat something one day and be fine, then eat it a week later and be extremely sick? The medical community answered with "It's IBS." I know the real answer now. It's because different brand names use different ingredients. One burger restaurant may add wheat, the other might not.

Though the years I developed other problems. Lethargy made me go back to the doctor and after blood tests, I was diagnosed with hypothyroid. The medication for this gave me more energy but did nothing for my IBS.

Scourge of my life. When I complained about having rough, blister-like breakouts on the back of my legs and arms I was told it was either eczema or winter dry skin. The recommendation was to use moisturizer and someone even told me to take vitamin E. None of this healed my skin but it did ease the breakouts a bit.

Since the IBS was an even bigger problem I pushed these stressful problems to the back of my mind and tried to find food I could eat. Everything now was making me sick. During one of my normal thyroid checkups I again mentioned the problems with my stomach. And the fact that even a plain old slice of bread made me nauseous. "How could that be?" I cried. "Bread was what you give to sick people!"

The doctor stopped and looked at me for a moment then told me about his mother who had celiac disease. He told me I probably didn't have it because of my weight (5 foot 6 inches and 160 pounds) and people with celiac disease are very thin. When I pressed him for more information he wrote down the name and told me to look it up on the Internet. He still doubted I had it.

At this point in my life I was desperate for an answer and I prayed to God everyday that he would send me a clue as to what was tormenting me. Could this be it? I logged onto my computer the first chance I got and started reading everything I could find on this disease.

I started looking into how many things in our everyday life contain gluten. Bread, cereals, pasta, pizza, and cakes were the obvious sources but I was soon to learn gluten is mixed into almost all processed foods. I immediately started a quest to get gluten out of my diet.

It was a lot harder than I ever suspected. Ninety percent of the soups, canned foods, and prepared foods on the market today contain gluten. It is used in some medicines, most sauces, spices (wheat flour is sometimes used to prevent clumping), modified food starch (food starch in the USA is suppose to be corn but when you add the word "modified" then wheat could be added), cough drops, stamps, and envelope glue. For a while it seemed like everything I looked at had gluten in it.

Another issue was cross-contamination. I needed to replace everything that could be hiding gluten including:

toasters, cutting boards, teflon pans, and plastic spatulas! It was incredibly depressing yet the more research I did the easier it got.

It definitely gets easier as time goes on. Within a month on a gluten-free diet my "IBS" and stomach cramps were gone!

People with celiac disease can live normal, healthy lives, and I found a lot of support on the Internet. There, people from all over the world join together to share hints, problems, and commiserate. It makes this whole diet thing more livable.

I went to my local health food store with a printout from a company that makes gluten-free foods and that now stocks a wide variety of gluten-free products. I'm finding pasta, breads, and even some cookies that are so good most people wouldn't know they are not made from "regular" flour. There are also several good mail order bakeries that have good bread, bagels, and other products made from rice, tapioca or potato flour. I order in quantity and freeze.

It definitely gets easier as time goes on. Within a month on a gluten-free diet my "IBS" and stomach cramps were gone! The nausea took a bit longer to improve but each day it was getting better.

When I returned to the doctor and said I believed I had celiac disease, he was doubtful. At my insistence he ordered the blood test. At that point I had been off of gluten for about six to eight weeks. The test was negative. By this time I had met other people with celiac disease though the Internet and they informed me the test would not be accurate unless I had been ingesting gluten for at least six weeks before the test. I double checked this information with some on-line celiac associations and it seems they were right.

My dilemma now was whether or not to go back on gluten for an accurate diagnosis. It was a hard decision. I have two daughters and I felt I needed to know since this could run in the family. My father suffered for years with gastrointestinal problems before dying at age 65 of colon cancer. I'm sure now he had celiac disease.

With that hanging over my head I decided to go back on gluten for answers. My first meal was a pizza! Yum! The next day I was fine. So I continued to eat gluten. Within two days the cramps and diarrhea were back. By two weeks I was sick everyday and having trouble getting myself to work, but I didn't give up. My husband thought I was crazy. He kept telling me I already knew what was

Would my tests have been positive if I had been tested before going gluten-free? I don't know and at this point I don't care. I know what makes me sick and I avoid it.

making me sick. Why was I doing this to myself? But I had made the decision to find out if I really had celiac disease so on I ate. On really bad days I took Imodium and sometimes didn't eat until I was safely home. The nausea was constant. Some days the cramping and pain was so bad I just couldn't eat at all. I don't know if this hurt my test results or not but there were times when I just couldn't bring myself to swallow any food at all. Eating caused the pain to worsen. I did this for six weeks.

The day of my blood test, I did not eat before I went to the lab at two in the afternoon. I was afraid if I ate anything at all I'd get sick at the lab and that would be too embarrassing. Ever sit in a room full of people while you were waiting for your turn, fighting nausea and just knowing everyone was watching when you got up to use the bathroom five times??? Let alone having to sit still long enough to get the blood drawn. The blood work all came back negative. At this point I had my sixteen-year-old daughter in for a blood test. The doctor thought I was crazy. She didn't fit the profile. I asked him to do it anyway to put my mind at ease and he did. The blood work was positive. Likewise my nineteen-year-old daughter tested positive. Both of them opted out of the endoscopes, even though this is thought to be the gold standard for diagnosis. They went gluten-free and are both feeling better on the diet.

Two weeks later I went for my endoscopy. I asked the gastroenterologist how many biopsies he was going to take and he told me, "Enough, don't worry." But I did worry. What if it's not enough? Celiac damage can be patchy and I desperately wanted an accurate diagnosis. The doctor called two days later and said the biopsy was fine.

So I am an undiagnosed celiac. I went gluten-free the day of my endoscopy and today I am feeling better than I have in my whole life! The "IBS" is gone, my skin is clearing and I never get nauseous. Today I feel healthy and I am living a much better life. Traveling still makes me nervous but it's getting easier as I learn to trust my body once again.

Would my tests have been positive if I had been tested before going gluten-free? I don't know and at this point I don't care. I know what makes me sick and I avoid it. It's as simple as that. I only wish I had understood that before going on the gluten challenge, it would have saved a lot of pain.

My biggest problem now is the people who say things like, "Oh, I couldn't live without pasta!" (Would they say to a diabetic, "I couldn't live without sugar"? (Of course not.) To these people I just say, "You could if it made you sick."

And I thank God everyday I have my answer: celiac disease. It's a different way of life but one that is quite livable. Pasta never tasted as good as being healthy feels.

An Unusual Discovery

by Valerie Bernes

I grew up in Lorain, Ohio, and earned a Bachelor of Music degree from the University of Cincinnati College Conservatory of Music. I played in a full-time professional orchestra for one year but found it was too stressful for me. So now I make my living as a secretary/administrative assistant and do music on the side. I also enjoy doing astrology and tarot readings.

In my mid-40's I was appalled by how fat I seemed to be getting, especially around the middle. Even strangers came up to me and asked if I was pregnant! I went on diets, but nothing ever seemed to help that midsection.

I think the way I discovered I had celiac disease was unusual. To be honest, I had never heard of it, but in 1997 I had a relationship with a man who, in short, dumped me for someone else. Looking back, I doubt it had anything to do with my body. At the time I felt devastated and thought it must be because I was "fat," so I decided to go on a starvation diet. For more than a week, all I had to eat was chicken broth (and the occasional piece of broccoli, celery or carrot). After that week, I was really feeling better.

Then, my stepfather invited me to a clambake. There, I ate those delicious clams in clam broth sopped up with, of course, bread. Well, the next day I felt awful and came to the conclusion I must be allergic to wheat (had still never heard of celiac disease). In my own naive way I began avoiding obvious foods with wheat and again felt better.

Over the years, with experimentation, I found the other toxic grains and slowly became aware of the incredible amount of processed foods that contain small amounts of these "poisons." For a number of years I could tolerate small amounts. I could still go to restaurants and eat things that didn't obviously contain wheat, rye, barley or oats.

That's no longer the case. About nine months ago I had to face the facts and go 100 percent gluten-free. That means no more restaurants and no more social life. At least going out. That was hard for me because I'm single.

In addition to the gluten intolerance my last bout with reactions left me lactose intolerant as well, at least for the time being. It's been a learning experience ever since. I have learned a lot about contamination in certain products (still haven't found any chips I can eat as snacks - potato or corn) and I avoid distilled vinegar. Some people are adamant that distilled vinegar is acceptable for celiacs, but I haven't found that to be the case. I'm not going to argue with them. Maybe it is for them, but is certainly isn't for me. People aren't all the same so why should celiacs be?

I am grateful God let me know about celiac disease and allowed me a few more years on this earth. I think my father had it, but never knew. He never stopped eating gluten and died from intestinal cancer at age 54. I am 53.

My hope is that more people become aware of this disease, especially food manufacturers, who could make our lives so much easier with appropriate labeling. And maybe, just maybe, some more restaurants might put a few gluten-free entrees on their menus (smile)!

Maintaining a gluten-free diet isn't easy in this gluten-saturated society, but it can be done. And it's definitely worth it if you have celiac disease.

New Celiac Disease Symptom: Reluctance To Get A Diagnosis

by Dimitrios Douros

Dimitrios has also written "Two Years Of Testing," which can be read earlier in this chapter.

The one thing that breaks my heart daily is the number of doctors reluctant to test for celiac disease in patients that have classic symptoms. Equally distressing is the number of patients that put up with such doctors and are timid to take the necessary steps to protect their health!

Recently, there was a message on the Listserv about a family whose daughter had many celiac disease symptoms. She was in the hospital with kidney problems, had eating disorders, and was skin-and-bones except for a bloated stomach. The doctor pushed back on the request to test for celiac disease even though a parent has already been diagnosed with it! The comment from the parents "... we will work with this doctor until he agrees to test for celiac disease."

So, today I want to register in the medical journals a new, often overlooked symptom of celiac disease:

NAME OF SYMPTOM:

Reluctance to Get a Diagnosis

DESCRIPTION OF SYMPTOM:

The reluctance to DEMAND a celiac panel (test) even though numerous celiac disease symptoms exist, have persisted for a period of time, have not been definitively linked to another medical condition and have not responded to any treatment.

TREATMENT:

Get up early in the morning, have a good breakfast, get the phone and Yellow Pages, sit in a comfortable chair, and call as many doctors as needed till you find one that knows the word CELIAC and is enthusiastic about testing you for it. Then make an appointment to be tested as soon as possible.

FOLLOW-UP:

a) Repeat treatment for any other family member and friend that has the same symptoms.

b) If you test positive, make sure your reluctant-to-test doctor knows and find a new doctor.

My Battle with Diabetes, Heart Disease, and Celiac

by Richard LeTourneau

My name is Richard (Dick) LeTourneau. I'm sixty years of age and live in Connecticut with Amanda, my wife of thirty-five years. Currently I am semi-retired and work part-time for a financial planner.

Approximately 25 years ago at the age of 35 I was diagnosed with type one, insulin independent, diabetes. That was unusual in and of itself since most type 1 diabetics are diagnosed when they are pre-teens. This meant years of insulin injections. Recently I went on the insulin pump which greatly simplifies my life. No syringes and no living my life by the clock.

About 11 years ago I started getting all kinds of "stomach problems." After a few years of reflux, stomach cramps and diarrhea, I went to a gastroenterologist. Because of my type 1 diabetes he diagnosed my problem as gastroparesis, a paralysis of the vegas nerve which controls the motility of food out of the stomach. He put me on Propulsid, which did nothing. The drug was eventually pulled by the FDA because it potentially caused heart problems. So, he prescribed another medication which made me sick. I came off it immediately.

A few years later I went to a second gastroenterologist who just loaded me up on prescription antacids and Tums. This helped somewhat, as long as I took three Tums every night before bed. Even then I'd occasionally wake up in the middle of the night with stomach acid in my mouth. Not a pleasant experience.

Approximately eight years ago I had quadruple coronary bypass surgery, probably due to the long term diabetes.

About a year ago my elbows broke out in very itchy, weepy sores. A dermatologist took two biopsies and sent them to a lab. They came back positive for dermatitis herpetiformis. The doctor explained you can't have dermatitis herpetiformis without celiac disease. I had never heard of either of them. So, off I went to a third gastroenterologist with my diagnosis of celiac disease in my hand. He did a blood test and ordered an endoscopy, which not surprisingly came back positive for celiac.

I guess the conclusion is that the patient has to be his own doctor. It seems my other conditions probably hindered my getting a proper diagnosis sooner. Some doctors go for the obvious and easy answer and don't scratch below the surface. They therefore could miss what else is wrong with you. Three doctors and eleven years later I finally received the correct diagnosis...strangely enough from a dermatologist. ✍

Alternative Medicine

by Valerie Wells

*I'm the mother of four adult sons, and grandmother of two. I
have a passion for health issues especially when it comes to diet and
natural approaches to healing. I work part time for an ear, nose and
throat surgeon, but my real "job" is volunteering my time and
energy to helping others find solutions for difficult health challenges.*

I'm a registered nurse with a conventional medical
background, but my experiences with conventional
and alternative medicine have caused me to become
passionate about "alternative" medicine. I suffered for ten
years with a mysterious illness that at times was erroneously
labeled fibromyalgia, depression, "stress," irritable bowel
syndrome, and I secretly suspect many doctors considered me
a hypochondriac.

Some years ago, I started a low carbohydrate diet for what
I self-diagnosed as carbohydrate intolerance. I got better.
When I reintroduced bread, I got worse. My doctor said, "So
don't eat bread." Gee thanks, doc. That visit was certainly
worth $60!

I began to investigate celiac disease. I attempted a gluten
challenge in preparation for a conventional celiac work up,

but was too ill to tolerate it for more than just a few days. Of course, my conventional testing for celiac disease came out negative. So I went ahead and ordered the complete gluten sensitivity panel from EnteroLab in Dallas, Texas.

> *Conventional medicine completely failed to help me, yet they are the ones who received the bulk of my health care dollars.*

Four physicians agreed that because EnteroLab tests revealed I carried two copies of the genes that predispose for celiac disease, and I can't tolerate gluten in any form, I probably had celiac disease. But since there's no "hard diagnostic evidence," I'm simply labeled "gluten intolerant."

Even after beginning the traditional gluten-free diet, I still did not recover fully. It took the help of a skilled naturopath and a year of intense "alternative" treatments to stop the downward spiral of my declining health. Conventional medicine completely failed to help me, yet they are the ones who received the bulk of my health care dollars.

I consider my life rescued by "alternative" medicine. I appreciate doctors who have the guts to follow their convictions regardless of peer approval. These are my heroes: people who have largely been rejected by their more conventional peers, are often called "quacks," suffered financial losses because of it, but have each in some way contributed to my family's healing and the healing of thousands of others. These are the REAL doctors who have broken the mold and learned to think outside of the rigid box of conventional medicine in order to become world class healers. Most conventional doctors will have a comfortable retirement, but the real healer's work and contribution to society lives on long after they are dead and buried.

When conventional medicine fails you, it's really valuable to have alternatives. In fact, most of us would probably be better off if we started out with alternative medicine in the first place! ✍️

Good News At Last

by Stephanie Murphy

I am 27 years old. I graduated from Colorado State University in 1998 with a Bachelors Degree in Animal Science. I developed an interest in the law shortly after graduation, and currently work as a Paralegal in Denver, Colorado. I have been married for four years. We do not yet have children. I enjoy competing in triathlons as well as training horses and horseback riding. I was diagnosed with celiac disease in September 2003 at the Mayo Clinic.

M y good luck changed to bad on June 29, 2002. It was during the run leg of a triathlon in Loveland, Colorado, at approximately mile 4 of 6.2. I felt a shooting pain in my right thigh, much different than the typical aches and pains well known to most runners. I continued running on it for about another mile, but around mile 5, the trusty endorphins I could always count on to get me through a race ran out. I fell to the ground in a heap of pain; my leg had given out. It was six weeks later that I found out I had suffered a stress fracture to the bone in my right thigh, every athlete's worst nightmare. Crutches in hand, I was prepared to sit on the bench for the four to six weeks it was supposed to take the stress fracture to heal.

Not only was the fracture not healed in six weeks, but the pain seemed to be getting worse and was spreading throughout my entire leg. I returned to my orthopedist seven months after the injury to ask why I was still in pain. I had several diagnoses ranging from a slow healing stress fracture to sciatica, but the diagnostic tests were all normal. I also found out around that time I had osteoporosis.

To most people, getting diagnosed with celiac disease might seem like a curse, but to me it has truly been a blessing.

I wondered why a 27-year-old woman would be getting osteoporosis, but my doctors had no answers for me. This was one of many unexplained medical conditions my doctors couldn't or wouldn't pay attention to. Others were a dramatic decrease in my vision during one particular year, and going two-and-a-half years without menstruating. I was told not menstruating was normal because I was exercising.

Finally, in March 2003, nine months after the injury, the fracture had finally healed, but my pain was getting worse. Any type of exercise was out of the question, including walking. I saw a physiatrist (a specialist in physical medicine), who ordered an MRI of my leg. Astonishingly, the MRI was completely normal. That doctor suggested I had RSD (reflex sympathetic dystrophy), a debilitating condition brought on by trauma that affects the sympathetic nervous system and promises a life of pain, misery and eventual confinement to a wheelchair.

By July 2003, my pain was so severe I was crippled into walking with a cane, and even that was excruciating. Truth be told, I probably should have been in a wheelchair, but I was too proud for that. Once an elite athlete I was now a chronic pain patient. The physiatrist had dumped me into a pain clinic because there was nothing else she could do with me. I was taking so many different pain medications I didn't know which end was up. I was still working full time, but only because my employer was too kind to let me go. I still had no diagnosis and every test that was run came back normal. In all of her infinite wisdom, the pain doctor concluded it was "in my head," and I "needed a psych consult." Granted I have problems, we all do, but I knew I wasn't crazy. I knew there was a reason for my pain so I decided to seek help from the Mayo Clinic.

On September 15, 2003, my husband and I flew to the Mayo Clinic in Scottsdale, Arizona. I gave my story to an internist, expecting her to be just like all the others, but I was shocked when she actually stopped and listened to me. Of course the leg pain was my chief concern, but I also mentioned I had been experiencing severe diarrhea and a 15 pound weight loss, which I chalked up to the pain medications. She immediately suspected sprue and ran the appropriate tests. It was not until my fifth day at Mayo that I finally got the good news: my diagnosis of celiac disease. Once I found out what celiac disease was and that it is completely manageable, I gave the internist a big hug. She seemed confused by my exultation and gratitude, so I tried to explain why I was so delighted.

To most people, getting diagnosed with celiac disease might seem like a curse, but to me it has truly been a blessing. I cannot explain the difference I feel in my body since getting the gluten out of my system. As an athlete, I have always had a keen awareness of my body and sense of self. I can say I feel like a new person, but that does not accurately describe the amazing changes that have taken place over the last six weeks. I have unleashed an energy I did not know I possessed, my skin has a brighter hue, and the depression that has hovered above me and followed me like a dark cloud for as long as I can remember has lifted.

Although my pain isn't completely gone, it's getting better every day thanks to a gluten-free diet. I'm weaning off of my pain medications, and I've even started swimming and riding my bike again. Racing triathlons may still be down the road a bit, but I'll get there soon. One thing I have learned in all of this is that time, nature, and patience are the three great healers. And getting rid of gluten doesn't hurt either!

Don't Give Up

by Stacie Collett

My name is Stacie Collett and for over a year I visited numerous doctors and endured multiple tests and procedures. I found myself feeling very discouraged and afraid I would never feel normal again. Finally after I was diagnosed with celiac disease I immediately began a gluten-free diet. The pain I suffered on a daily basis disappeared and I am feeling better than I have in a long time.

After suffering terribly for over a year with nausea, diarrhea, cramps, abdominal pain, audible bowel sounds, fatigue, headaches, hair loss, and significant weight loss as well as other symptoms, I was finally diagnosed with celiac disease.

My story begins when I first visited a gastroenterologist who thought I had a severe case of irritable bowel syndrome in my small intestines. While reviewing my test results with him we discussed the possibility of celiac disease. He insisted that since my blood work came back normal a biopsy would also be normal. I mentioned going gluten-free and his response was it is a hard diet to stick to. He insisted it had to be irritable bowel syndrome, or maybe it could be a parasite. So he gave me a prescription for a powerful antibiotic in case it was a parasite and sent me on my way again. I walked out of his office very discouraged, feeling no one cared and feeling I would never feel normal again. I suffered with so much pain I just wanted a name to put with my symptoms. At least something I could find a way of fighting. Something I could do to prevent the symptoms from recurring.

During the past year the thought of feeling normal again was becoming an unattainable dream instead of a possibility. I could not even remember what it felt like to "feel good." I withdrew from my family and friends and did not attend any social functions. I always wanted to stay home but then I felt guilty because I was causing my husband and two children to suffer right along with me. However, through all of this my family has been very supportive.

After my year of suffering and persistence in trying to find out what was wrong, I finally received my celiac diagnosis. I was very excited to finally find out my problems had a name and even more excited because I knew how to correct it. I found an awesome support group on the Internet that has helped me tremendously. I can relate exactly to what other celiacs are going through. I felt relieved to find such a place to ask questions, voice my concerns and to know there was a possibility of helping others going through the same things I have been going through. I am happy to say I have been gluten-free for about a month. After only a couple of days I could actually feel a difference in myself. The unattainable dream of feeling normal is finally becoming a reality and it's wonderful!

It has been a challenge to find foods I can eat but it's one I will gladly accept especially knowing how much better I feel on the gluten-free diet.

If you think you may have celiac disease please do not let the doctors tell you any different. With so many doctors out there not celiac knowledgeable, it is misdiagnosed every single day. Only you know how and what you are feeling and what is normal and not normal for your body. Do not give up; keep researching until you find the answers you are looking for.

Good luck! ✍

Celiac: An Inherited Disease

Why Couldn't You Just Leave Me The House?

*There's a family history of sprue,
I guess I should be tested too.
My health is okay,
But I'll test anyway.
Surprise, I tested positive, it's true.*

It's In Our Genes

by Frances Monteith

I am the mother of four children. Three of my children have celiac disease. I was diagnosed in 1999, a year after my fourth child was born. We are all healthy and doing well on the diet.

When our daughter Lauren was diagnosed with celiac disease in 1996, we were told it was genetic, and that my husband Greg and I should be tested. Since neither of us had any symptoms at the time, we put this information in the back of our minds as a "someday" thing we must do and went on with our lives.

Our next child, Danny, was born a robust and healthy baby, but soon after we began introducing cereals and whole foods into his diet, we discovered that he, too, had celiac disease. Still, Greg and I procrastinated about having ourselves tested. We moved from New York to New Jersey, and with reasons of new medical insurance, yearly deductibles, and every other excuse under the sun, we delayed the testing further.

Our focus changed when the Westchester support group announced a conference that would include serum testing of first-degree relatives as part of a University of Maryland prevalence study. Now there were no excuses. We attended

My older sister and my mother were also completely asymptomatic. Yet they all have celiac disease.

the conference in September 1997, and as we waited in line for our blood to be drawn, Greg and I chided each other: "It's going to be you." "No, it's going to be you!" I was five months pregnant with our fourth child, and was so sure it wasn't me that I placed a wager on Greg's blood test results.

I lost the bet. On the day I was discharged from the hospital after giving birth, I received my blood test results. I had elevated IgG and IgA levels, and would need to be biopsied for celiac disease. My biopsy then was inconclusive but a year later I did receive a definite diagnosis.

But this was only the beginning. Being one of nine children myself, I called all of my siblings and my parents, and asked them to please consider being tested. It took some coaxing to get past a lot of "It can't be us, we're all so healthy." I convinced seven family members to go to the next blood screening conducted by the Westchester group and lo and behold, three of my family members had positive blood test results. Their follow-up biopsies confirmed the diagnosis of celiac disease.

My dad is 72 years old, six-feet tall, weighs well over 200 pounds and was feeling well. My older sister and my mother were also completely asymptomatic. Yet they all have celiac disease. Recently, my father-in-law was diagnosed unexpectedly with celiac disease while having another procedure done during an endoscopy.

Needless to say, we had been surprised to find celiac disease on both sides of my family, but we were now amazed to find it on my husband's side of the family as well. The point I want to make is, once a family member has been diagnosed, please encourage all first-degree relatives to be serum tested. Now my father's brother, who has been ill for years, is starting to wonder if this is the answer to many of his health problems. He has agreed to be tested. Several of my cousins are piecing together their own health stories, and are getting tested. My brother, though his antibodies were negative, is highly symptomatic and he is being biopsied this summer. The ball is rolling, and maybe many lives will be saved.

How Can I Have Celiac?
I Have No Symptoms
by Amy Kravitz

I currently work as a children's services librarian at the Westfield New Jersey Memorial Library. My husband and I reside in Morganville, New Jersey. I would like to give special thanks to my mother, Arleen Dresnack, for all of her support this past year. I would also like to thank Diane Paley, the head of the Central New Jersey CSA/USA Celiac Support Group for encouraging family members of those with celiac sprue to be screened.

I am basically a healthy, 31-year-old female. My younger brother has had celiac sprue since he was an infant. He had the classic symptoms of celiac disease and was lucky to be diagnosed rather quickly at a specialized hospital in New York City.

My brother has never known from eating bread, pizza, or even Dunkin' Donuts. I give him a lot of credit because in his 28 years, I can never remember hearing him complain about his disease. He just accepted celiac disease as his lot in life and went on living. I remember back to our childhood days when he had birthday parties, school parties, and family parties to attend. My mother always helped him out by preparing foods he could eat. Back in those years I can remember myself thinking, "Boy, do I feel sorry for Michael. I'm glad I don't have to contend with what he does."

As a result of my brother's condition, my mother is active in a local celiac support group. About two years ago her support group encouraged all of its members to screen first-degree relatives of people who had celiac disease. My mother wanted herself, my father, and me to be tested to rule out the possibility we had celiac disease. At the time I was newly married, feeling well, and happily employed. I wanted nothing to do with this illness called celiac disease. My family figured if anyone had celiac disease it would be my father as he has some digestive problems.

I can still vividly remember the day of the celiac screening. It was on a rainy Sunday, and we had to drive for over two hours to a hospital in Tarrytown, New York. My parents and I had blood taken that day, and I never gave celiac sprue a second thought.

I went back to living my life, when one day my parents called with some surprising news. They tested negative for celiac disease, whereas I tested positive! I was in total shock! How could someone like me come out positive for this disease? The only possible symptom I had was constipation, but I figured that was just the way my body worked.

For about a year I was in denial of the whole thing. I even told my mom never to mention the "C" word again! If I felt fine, why would I give up foods I loved? I was always eating out, and I especially enjoyed fast foods and ethnic restaurants.

My mother kept on my case. She insisted I get screened again for confirmation of my diagnosis, and I begrudgingly went. Sure enough, the second test reconfirmed the first. I had celiac sprue.

After the second round of results came back the diagnosis weighed more heavily on my mind. I originally thought celiac disease was a wheat allergy. I started to do some research and found out celiac sprue is an autoimmune disease which could have serious complications if one didn't adhere to the diet. I also found out virtually asymptomatic people like myself can have the same bodily devastation as people with symptoms. The only way to prevent this would be to adopt the gluten-free diet. I thought long and hard on this. Someday I would like to have a family and this was one of my main reasons for going on the diet.

Although I didn't feel that way originally, I am now thankful to my mother for pursuing a diagnosis for me. If it weren't for the birth of my brother and my mother's encouragement, I would probably never have known I have celiac.

My mother has been very supportive since my diagnosis. She took me on my first trip to the supermarket to show me what I could eat and how to read labels. That was a very difficult day for me as my life was suddenly narrowed down to a very small list of foods. Nevertheless, she helped me out.

It has now been approximately eight months since I've been on the gluten-free diet. I am at the stage where I am adjusting to this new lifestyle, and my mother has always been by my side helping. She often buys me pastries from a gluten-free bakery thirty miles away. Last week she made many gluten-free dishes for my brother and me to eat when we were invited elsewhere for Thanksgiving dinner.

It has been a year of surprise and change for me. I am

doing well on the diet, and still learning things. I know the diet is working because my one symptom, constipation, has gone away. I am now involved in on-line celiac support groups as well as a local support group. This has been a tremendous help and I recommend everyone with celiac disease get involved in a group.

Although I didn't want to acknowledge it at first, I am very grateful to my mother for caring enough about me to have me diagnosed and for assisting me through a trying first year with a new condition and a brand new lifestyle.

An initial diagnosis of celiac sprue disease can be downright scary and unsettling, but with the help of a good support network, things will get easier. ✍

The Story Of A Family

by Mitzi Berkhout

My celiac disease was diagnosed in 1990. I wondered how many people in my area had the disease so I started a support group. It was named The West MI Celiac Support Group #78, Chapter of the CSA/USA. At our first meeting we had 55 people and of them 35 were celiacs who thought they were the only one with celiac disease.

When I was finally diagnosed with celiac disease in 1990 I had no idea what this disease was, or how it would change my life forever. I read everything I could on the subject, but there was not much out there for the layperson. I didn't know it was genetic or I had a distant relative who also had celiac disease. So, how do I know my great-grandmother had this disease? It was a twist of fate that led me to this discovery!

While searching in libraries, I read a book from England on celiac disease. The book explained, in the old days, celiac disease was called the "wasting disease." A light went off in my head!! My grandmother had told me her mother, whose name was Mary Adams, had died from the "wasting disease" in 1872 when she was only 32 years old. She left behind her husband, Will, and their three children, one of whom was my grandmother. Five years later Will died of tuberculosis leaving the children orphans. My grandmother and her brother and sister had grown up in an orphanage in Pennsylvania.

I often think of Mary, whose celiac disease I inherited. She was young and didn't know exactly what was wrong with her, but she knew she was very ill and barely able to take care of her family. In letters to his children, written after Mary died, Will relates how really sick Mary was even long before my grandmother was born. At that time they didn't know what caused her disease, much less how to treat it. Will said some of her relatives had the disease too. We know that celiac disease is genetic, but in those days they didn't know much about genetics. However, Will's account of Mary's illness fits the disease we call celiac disease.

My grandmother had stomach trouble all her life. When she was a young woman, she had surgery to have part of her intestines removed. When I was a young girl, I remember my grandmother always being on a diet and that everything bothered her stomach. She was a little woman and always very thin. When she died, she had cancer in her intestines.

Now that I am a celiac and know more about the disease, I would say my mother was also a celiac. She had a bloated stomach and was sometimes heavy, sometimes slim. She had signs of celiac disease but was never diagnosed. She was also an insulin-dependent diabetic. She died of congestive heart failure, unrelated to celiac disease.

In my family, I had two brothers that had insulin-dependent diabetes. One of them had celiac disease. When my daughter died in a car crash, an autopsy revealed she too had celiac disease. My other daughter, who has had diabetes since age six, does not have celiac disease.

There are several cousins on the same blood line that also have diabetes, and one cousin with celiac disease. So far, my grandchildren do not have celiac disease, but I'm watching them very closely and I've encouraged them to be tested.

I hope something will be discovered in the future so that generations of yet unborn people will be free of this disease. In the meantime, I encourage anyone who has someone with celiac disease in their family be tested. It does run in the family. ✍

I Should Have Known

by Lynn Pipher

I am a 46-year-old woman who pressed my doctors to find out what was wrong with me. After eight years of suffering, I was finally diagnosed with celiac disease in November 2000. I live just outside of Ontario, Canada, and am married with two sons. I work full time in a busy law firm and manage to maintain a gluten-free diet. My hope in sharing my story is to give anyone else wondering what's wrong with them some insight into this ever increasing condition. It makes you want to ask: "What's in that wheat, anyway?"

Before I became sick, my father was very ill and died from complications of celiac disease. He was only 66. He developed non-Hodgkin's lymphoma which is something that COULD happen if celiac disease is left untreated. Once he was finally diagnosed, he adopted a gluten-free diet but it was too late. By then his system was already affected by our poison: GLUTEN.

So, you might ask, "Why didn't you realize what was wrong with you once the diarrhea started increasing in severity and occurrence?" I don't know. It was a hectic time. My second child had just been born. I read somewhere that a pregnancy can trigger celiac disease but I didn't put all the pieces together. My family flew to Texas from Toronto,

Canada, to introduce my new son to my sister and her family. That's where it all began. I actually thought I had traveler's diarrhea due to the water. It was so severe that a whole box of Imodium didn't help it a bit. Upon my return I went to my doctor and he ran some tests. No virus and no parasites. He said I was fine.

The diarrhea came and went, but with a young family and working full time, I just tried to keep up with my routine. I started researching and talking to as many people who would talk to me about something so personal. An herbalist gave me a mixture of bran to put in my orange juice in the morning. That made me sicker. Often, I would turn to toast as comfort food as I thought it wouldn't be so hard on my stomach. Toast equals gluten and it just made my condition worse.

Two years after Texas, I continued to have unrelenting diarrhea. To make matters worse, I found a lump in my breast. I had a lumpectomy. The tissues were biopsied and they were found to be cancerous so I was scheduled for chemotherapy and radiation. The diarrhea continued. I asked my oncologist about it and he gave me a tiny little pill that paralyzed my colon for a few days. That was not a very good idea. I have always felt I ended up with breast cancer due to my compromised immune system from my celiac disease, although no doctor would agree with my theory.

As time went by, I learned to live with what the doctors had labeled irritable bowel syndrome. I accepted this diagnosis but there were more problems besides the diarrhea. My leg muscles were weak and sore, my joints inflamed, I was always tired and my brain was in a constant fog. I couldn't think straight and I was depressed. I needed a lot of dental work, lost teeth, and my gums got terribly red and inflamed. My system was malnourished.

My family doctor was aware of my family history, but when I approached the subject, he kept telling me the biopsy for the diagnosis of celiac disease would be "the last thing we tried." In the fall of 2000 (eight years after my trip to Texas), I finally demanded "the" biopsy from my family doctor and he sent me to

I knew I did not want the same thing that happened to my father to happen to me so I started a gluten-free diet the next day. I'm glad I did.

a gastroenterologist. The biopsy proved without a doubt I had celiac disease, no question about it.

The day I got my diagnosis I cried. My specialist told me there was nothing to cry about. I didn't have colon cancer and I could easily manage the disease by watching what I ate. I cried because there was something else bothering me. Not only did I feel a terrible sense of loss that I'd have to dramatically change my diet and lifestyle, but I was also thinking about my father. This same disease killed him at too young an age.

I knew I did not want the same thing that happened to my father to happen to me, so I started a gluten-free diet the next day. I'm glad I did. It changed my health and outlook. I began researching about the disease so I could be more empowered. Because of the information I learned, I asked my family doctor for a bone density test. I wanted to be checked for two reasons. First, I went through menopause when I was 37 years old (this was chemically induced by the chemo) and I discovered that without estrogen, bones become more porous. The second reason was I found out that the villi in the intestines are the way nutrients are absorbed from your food to your blood. With celiac disease, those villi are flattened by the immune response to gluten and nutrients and minerals aren't absorbed properly. I'm glad I requested

My brother and sister both take antidepressants. They don't think they have celiac disease and refuse the test because they both say "But I don't have diarrhea."

the test since it showed I had osteoporosis. I started taking the drug Fosamax. This together with calcium supplementation, exercise and increased dairy intake is starting to reverse the damage. I learned I had to take charge of my own health rather than leave it in the hands of my doctors. Some people are faster learners than others.

Through a gluten-free diet, my mental health has improved as well. The brain fog, memory scramble, fatigue and depression lifted weeks into the diet. The inability for my intestines to absorb vital nutrients, vitamins and minerals is the reason I was so fatigued and depressed.

Being forced to eat gluten-free was a blessing in disguise. Celiacs all eat so much better than the general population in North America. I'd be lying if I said this diet was easy to conquer. But it is one that is well worth your good health. It was very difficult at first, walking through a food court wondering what in the world I could eat. Everything in our modern society is either breaded, on a bun or "Do you want anchovies on that?" Food is central to our society and socially, it is a huge adjustment. Office "pizza" parties or finding gluten-free items on menus are daunting.

My husband became an instant ingredient label reader and my advocate. He speaks to grocery managers to see why a certain gluten-free food is not on the shelf or to waitresses to ensure what I am eating is free from what makes me so sick.

One post on my celiac Web group changed how I look at my diet. The poster wrote about the deprivation celiacs feel. He said it's time we look at what we CAN eat, not what we CANNOT eat. I took his words to heart and that's how I cope with this diet. I will maintain it for life as I'd like to get to know my grandchildren once my two boys (Alex is 15 and Eric is 12) decide to have families of their own. They are fully aware of what celiac is so should they develop problems in the future, they will NOT allow eight years to go by without a test.

Research indicates that approximately 1 in 133 people have this disease. Many don't know it. It hides under the guise of other illnesses. Sometimes people with celiac disease are anemic as iron is not absorbed. My brother and sister both take antidepressants. They don't think they have celiac disease and refuse the test because they both say, "But I don't have diarrhea." I think I too was in the same denial state for my eight years of suffering.

My father did say to me once, "If you ever get unrelenting diarrhea, have it checked out." but I didn't recall that conversation until the pieces were put together. Hindsight is 20/20.

I should have known. ✐

Have Your Family Tested

by Shelly Hampton

I was diagnosed with celiac in 2002, after a two-and-a-half year decline in my health. I am the mother of three children and our family lives in Delaware.

At the time of my diagnosis in 2002, I had lost a third of my body weight because of loss of appetite, and was pretty much homebound because I was so ill.

After my diagnosis, I learned as much about celiac disease as possible. I wanted to get better and live a long, healthy life. One of the things I learned was the importance of siblings being tested for celiac disease. I provided information to my brother and sister and encouraged them to ask for a blood test.

About 10 months after my diagnosis, my sister mentioned it to her doctor. His response was that since celiac was so rare, if one person in the family had it, it was very unlikely another one would. I couldn't believe what she was telling me. Didn't the doctor know celiac disease runs in families? Didn't he know that since I had it, it was more likely, not less likely that my sister might have it? I know she didn't push the matter, so

I supplied her with articles about the disease and again stressed the importance of testing.

Another year passed, and again I stressed the importance to my brother and sister of getting tested for celiac disease. I know no one wants to have celiac disease, but the fact is whether or not you admit you have it, the damage is still being done to your body. I stressed to them I didn't want them to go through what I went through and I didn't want them to die because they were not tested. I told them if the test comes back negative, I wouldn't bring it up again.

My sister is particularly the one I'm worried about. She's borderline diabetic, has high blood pressure along with the classic symptoms of celiac disease and generally feels rotten overall. When she recently went to the doctor, she again mentioned being tested for celiac disease. Once again, he explained how rare a disease it was, and if she insisted on being tested, he'd order the test, but couldn't justify it to insurance.

It's very frustrating that doctors still think celiac disease is a rare disease. It affects so many and in so many different ways. Even though I didn't have classic symptoms, I know if I had been tested for it in the beginning, insurance would have been spared the cost of sending me to 14 different doctors, repeated CT scans, MRI's, and so many other costly tests.

I know that my sister doesn't want to have this disease. Who does? One uninformed doctor passing on bad information can undo the work of those of us who are trying our best to educate our family. As long as there are doctors insisting on celiac being a rare disease, the patient would rather believe the doctor and not be tested. ✍

Joining the Celiac Life

by Janet McMillan

I have been married to John for over 40 years. Originally from New Zealand, we have lived in Brisbane, Australia for the last seven years. We have four children: Nigel, Anna, Kate and Andrew and 11 grandchildren. Kate and her daughter, Amelia, both have celiac disease.

My husband John teaches guitar, religious education and sings barbershop. I am too busy being wife, mother and grandmother to do much else, but I love reading, gardening and of course, now, learning all I can on gluten-free cooking.

For years John had suffered with rashes, three broken ankles and dystonia, which is a neurological condition that affects his right arm. Doctors could not explain the rashes or why he kept breaking his ankles, apart from the fact his bone density scan showed weakness in the hips.

Our daughter, Kate, and her daughter, Amelia, had been diagnosed with celiac disease and Kate kept saying that one of us must have it. Knowing I had cousins who were wheat intolerant, I went and had the blood test. The results showed a slight intolerance to wheat. So I thought, "Oh well it must be me."

But Kate is nothing if persistent and said Dad had to have tests too. So John had the blood test and he was off the scale. We then each went through a biopsy and mine was totally clear but John's was a disaster.

Yes, there is grieving, not only from the one with it but the partner too. Our life style had to change dramatically but I was the one who had to make the change as far as the food and cooking went. Shopping took twice as long. I took out all the books the library had on gluten-free cooking to learn as much as I could and to have options. Then came the cleaning out of the pantry and cupboards. My friends didn't mind. They benefited as I gave a lot away. I love to cook so you can imagine what I had in that pantry.

The change is now complete. We just had our first gluten-free Christmas and it was great. Kate is so sweet, she had a gift box of gluten-free food sent to us.

John is 65 this year, so you can imagine what a change it has been for him, but he says he wouldn't know he was eating gluten-free as I have done it so well. I cook lots of my normal recipes using gluten-free products. Because we live on a pension I have found the food bills are much dearer as for some reason everyone thinks if it is gluten-free it should cost twice as much.

John plays the guitar and has struggled over the last 10 years because of the dystonia. In the last three weeks he has begun to play pieces he has not been able to play for 20 years, so we wonder if the dystonia and celiac disease have some connection.

We have suggested to all family members that they have the test. John is one of 13, but like many people the attitude is "no, we couldn't have that." A great thing out of this is our family doctor is now sending a lot more of her patients for blood tests for celiac disease.

I think one of the things that stops people from investigating if maybe they have celiac disease is the fear of the changes to their lifestyle if it's diagnosed. We were probably less than sympathetic to Kate when she was diagnosed. But she is certainly much healthier and because she did all the hard work, we have been able to incorporate it all into our lives very easily.

Welcome to the world of the celiacs. ✍️

Janet's daughter, Kate, has written "Welcome To The World of Celiac Disease," which can be read in Chapter Three and her granddaughter, Amelia, has written "I Miss Oreo Biscuits," which can be read in Chapter Four.

My New Life

Wheat No More, My Baby

> They told me I couldn't eat wheat,
> It seemed an overwhelming feat.
> Throw the pizza away,
> No bread for today.
> But the payoff, I'm feeling upbeat.

Welcome To The World Of Celiac Disease

by Kathryn Dani

My name is Kathryn (Kate) and I'm 36 and married with three wonderful children. My father, my daughter and myself all have celiac disease. It actually makes it easier at family gatherings as we make sure everything is gluten-free. I live in Australia but am New Zealand born and from good Irish/Scottish stock (far more chance of getting celiac disease with that bloodline).

Before I tell my story let me share these thoughts with you. I have found celiac disease is not the end of the world but the beginning of a new life and better health. One of the things I found most helpful to me when I was diagnosed was joining on-line support groups and my local celiac society. Their help has been invaluable. The on-line support groups are fantastic because with so many odd things that can happen to you when you have celiac disease, you can be guaranteed you'll find someone out there who has the same symptom or has gone through the same thing. It is important not to feel alone and the groups help that tremendously. We share recipes, places to eat out, and just generally support each other.

For those that are not diagnosed or are just gluten intolerant, the on-line sites are great for you too. I know that many of you found out you could not eat gluten by trial and error and that there is nothing on this earth that will make you eat gluten again just to get a diagnosis. This is where these groups are great. So do not alienate yourselves. Join a community and enjoy friendship and great advice from people who have trod the path before you.

> *My local doctor told mum to sew mothballs to the bottom of my dresses and that would help. It only helped in losing friends!*

Now, for my story.

When I turned 33 my world felt like it was falling apart. My health was gone and I felt as if my mind was leaving me as well. I thought this was the start of something terrible. But in fact, as it turned out, the worst was nearing the end, not the beginning.

The beginning was when I was a child and had anemia. No one knew why, so I was given tablets to take and had multiple blood tests. My mother would give me a spoonful of malt each day to build me up. I would wake crying during the night with terrible leg cramps and my dad would massage my legs until I went back to sleep. My local doctor told mum to sew mothballs to the bottom of my dresses and that would help. It only helped in losing friends! I often complained of a "sore tummy" but that was put down to attention seeking and trying to get out of school. These problems continued without relief.

When I turned 22, I had the most severe pain in my gut just below my sternum. Off I went to the doctors who told me I was stressed and had a stomach ulcer. More tablets were given but no tests were undertaken. Often at night I couldn't sleep because of what I call "sugar legs." I felt like I constantly had to move them and couldn't keep them still. It was so bad that I often had to sleep with my legs up against a wall.

By the time I was 33, along with everything else, I was suffering muscle twitches and terrible bowel cramps. I was so tired all the time I just wanted to sleep and I had turned into a fisher woman. (For those not familiar with the term, imagine a woman with her hair in rollers, in an apron, holding a rolling pin over her head. She is screaming and yelling at her poor helpless husband or kids for some minor mistake that they may have made. She is unpleasant to be around and is a bit of a nag. It is the biggest insult to be called a fisher woman. It's a bit like a slap in the face.) It did not take much to set me off. My head felt fuzzy and befuddled and it made me feel so helpless. I couldn't think straight. My eyelids often felt heavy, and if I could have, I would have used toothpicks to prop them open (however that wasn't an option). I started having flooding once a month with terrible cramps to go with it.

On doing the rounds of the doctors I was told I had irritable bowel syndrome, chronic fatigue, a stomach ulcer and yes, let's take your uterus out.

As a last resort I went to a naturopath. Straight away she felt my problem was gluten and that I should go off it. I was willing to try anything by this stage as I felt I was only surviving, not living. So I went off gluten and six months later I felt as if I had been reborn. My muscle twitches and sugar legs had gone. So too the irritable bowel, stomach ulcer, chronic fatigue, heavy bleeding, and mood swings. It was the most amazing feeling. I cancelled the hysterectomy as it was no longer needed.

It is easy to stick to the diet as I know the consequences if I don't. As more people are being diagnosed, it is becoming easier to eat out. You do learn to adapt. I still have times when I crave fresh white bread or Kentucky Fried Chicken but it passes.

Celiac disease can seem frightening, bewildering and a huge lifestyle change. But believe me, when you feel better, when you function normally again without pain and all the other associated problems, you will be so glad you know what is wrong. Of all the diseases you can have, this is the best. No injections, no medications, and you can live a normal healthy life by following the diet. Good luck to all of you.

Kate's mother, Janet McMillan, has written "Joining The Celiac Life," which can be read in Chapter Two and her daughter, Amelia, has written "I Miss Oreo Biscuits," which can be read in Chapter Four.

A New Life For Our Son

by Valerie Wells

Valerie has also written "Alternative Medicine," which can be read in Chapter One.

My husband and I were the proud parents of a beautiful baby boy 26 years ago. George was found to be of above average intelligence but was considered an underachiever with attention deficit disorder all through school. By the time he was in high school he was constantly complaining of "brain strain" and could barely cope with the rigors of academic life. We withdrew him from public school and he graduated from a state approved home school program. He was determined to further his education and enrolled in community college but his grades steadily declined in spite of all his best efforts. He found it impossible to concentrate on many of his subjects, especially math and was put on academic probation.

During his time off from school, he was very depressed, chronically fatigued and diagnosed with fibromyalgia. His condition continued to deteriorate until he became tormented by both visual and auditory hallucinations.

About this time, I was diagnosed "gluten intolerant." I

wondered if gluten sensitivity could be at the root of George's problems. I delicately, gently talked him into conventional blood tests for celiac disease, but they came out "negative." My next step in handling this difficult situation was to get him to submit to a mouth swab for a gene test and to donate a stool sample for testing through EnteroLab. This was no easy task since his behavior was so unpredictable. He did, however, cooperate. His gene test revealed two copies of the gene and his stool test came out positive for "gluten sensitivity with malabsorption," Dr. Kenneth Fine's equivalent to celiac disease.

My son reluctantly started the gluten-free diet and all his demons vanished, the burdening fatigue and depression lifted and his muscle pain eventually melted away. His social life blossomed and, best of all, his hallucinations stopped. He was suddenly a happy young man able to control his behavior and hopeful for a bright future. He re-enrolled in school and to his utter delight found a focus on math and science that he had never had. He enjoyed his new role as the "smart guy" and became his classmates' favorite study buddy. His college algebra teacher even hired George to be his assistant.

He was so happy with his new life, he composed two enchanting songs for the piano, "Gratitude" and "Happily Ever After." George managed to improve his grades and was accepted to a four year university where he is now pursuing his dream: a bachelor's degree in history. He's now living a normal life (except for the gluten-free diet) which was something no one thought would be possible three years ago when he couldn't even hold a job.

Had we relied on the results of his negative blood test and not delved further, he'd still be sick, labeled schizophrenic or bipolar and would have been put on psychotropic medications for life. I'm sure he'd never succeed in college in that condition.

He has done his best to follow the gluten-free diet for over two years now. My husband and I consider the gluten-free diet a miracle that saved our son's future. ✐◻

Living With Celiac Disease: Our First Year

by Sue Clayton

I was diagnosed with celiac disease in October 2002. My husband, two children and brother all have celiac disease. I am the Branch Manager for the Gluten-Free Group of Arizona.

J ust about a year ago, I tested positive for celiac disease. During the last twelve months, every one of my family members (I mean, those who have been willing to be tested) have also tested positive. These include my son (age nine), daughter (age six), husband, mother-in-law and brother. A year ago, I knew nothing about gluten and spent as little time as possible in the kitchen. Today, I'm an experienced gluten-free cook and spend a great deal of my time preparing food.

It's easy to remember those horrible first few months of the gluten-free lifestyle. I was diagnosed just three days before I had emergency gallbladder surgery and spent my first few weeks living on Ensure, Snickers bars and potato chips. I was overwhelmed, frustrated, and depressed. I tried many of the gluten-free products at local health food stores (particularly breads) and they were awful. I also ordered many mail order products. Not only were they expensive, they tasted terrible.

Six weeks later, my son was diagnosed. All of a sudden I needed more than a diet of meal replacement shakes and junk food. Trips to the grocery store took forever as I read labels and abandoned our favorite foods. Purchasing school lunches was suddenly out of the question.

> *For the first two weeks, she came home crying almost every day when she couldn't eat birthday cake, donuts, or candy. How I wished I could take away her pain!*

I'd wake up every morning with the panicked thought: "What am I going to feed Kevin today?"

Fortunately, two wonderful things happened around this time. The first was attending LynnRae Ries' cooking classes at the Gluten-Free Cooking School in Phoenix. It was a pleasure to see smiling faces enjoying gluten-free cooking and gluten-free living. The food was delicious and after a short time, things didn't seem quite so daunting. I am continually amazed at LynnRae's creativity, and I have learned to make some delicious gluten-free dishes. I also enjoy the camaraderie from these cooking classes.

The second blessing was the formation of the Southeast Valley R.O.C.K. (Raising Our Celiac Kids) Group. Our first meeting was a cookie exchange. After weeks of saying "No Kevin, you can't eat that," we were greeted with a lovely Christmas table filled with gluten-free goodies. I choked back tears when my son looked incredulously at the table and asked, "Are you sure I can eat anything I want?" Kevin was also able to make friends with other celiac kids, which was great because now he didn't feel so alone. Other parents generously shared their sources for delicious (or at least tolerable) gluten-free substitutes and mail order shopping became easier. Since then we have enjoyed many wonderful R.O.C.K. events and I am very grateful for the wisdom shared during our meetings.

When Angie was diagnosed in April, just after her sixth birthday, I thought my heart would break. With the gluten-free logistics in place, I mourned the plans I'd had for both of my children. How would we travel? Could they stay over at a friend's house? Would they be able to go to an out of state university? Certainly, they could never live in residence. Angie wondered if she'd ever find a husband who would accept celiac disease and allow a gluten-free kitchen.

In addition, kindergarten at Angie's school used many food related rewards. For the first two weeks, she came home crying almost every day when she couldn't eat birthday cake, donuts, or candy. How I wished I could take away her pain!

At that point I signed up to attend the Gluten Intolerance Group's June 2003 conference in Denver. This was a wonderful experience on many levels. I met fabulous people, tasted some delicious food and got a real understanding of the medical issues surrounding celiac disease. I also heard many horror stories from people about the length of time it took them (or their children) to be diagnosed, and how sick they had to become before celiac was considered as the problem. I came away from that conference feeling empowered about celiac disease and ready to get on with our lives.

When my husband was diagnosed in July, we faced many different challenges. To begin with, he had to start bringing his lunch instead of eating in the office cafeteria. Mark's job also requires lots of lunch meetings and travel. He's learned to pack Ensure for plane rides and breakfasts, and to look for an Outback Steakhouse for meals on his own. So far, his colleagues have been great about choosing restaurants where there are gluten-free choices. At local restaurants Mark will call ahead and

> *Mostly though, living with celiac disease doesn't seem that terrible. It is inconvenient, for sure, but I try to keep it in perspective.*

explain his restrictions. If lunch (usually pizza or sandwiches) is brought into the office, Mark will drink soda and eat a meal replacement bar.

Recently, I spent a week at a facility that serves only raw foods. I was excited not to have to deal with my dietary restrictions and to enjoy raw fruits and vegetables. To my horror, a significant portion of the diet came from sprouted wheat and from a drink made of fermented wheat sprouts. The director of the program insisted celiacs could eat wheat sprouts because the sprouting process removes the gluten. This was the policy of the facility and it was very difficult experience.

Mostly though, living with celiac disease doesn't seem that terrible. It is inconvenient, for sure, but I try to keep it in perspective. We eat a lot of meat and vegetables, which enables me to shop at regular stores. I've discovered some delicious gluten-free baking mixes and have made baking a part of my routine. I've accepted we can't travel anywhere that doesn't have a kitchen unit. When we drove to San Diego for a week this summer, we rented a unit with a kitchenette and brought along mixes, pots, my KitchenAid mixer and a microwave. Not exactly traveling light but it worked! The kids have gluten-free treat boxes in the classroom and parents are generally good about accommodating our dietary issues.

I often feel like I've been thrown back into a time before convenience and fast food dominated our lives. To be honest, I miss those days and still resent the amount of time involved in food preparation. For everyone else, however, the change is a positive one. Instead of cheeseburgers at school, my children now enjoy nutritious lunches with homemade chocolate chip cookies. My husband loves taking home-cooked lunches and doesn't miss the miserable menus at his office. I've taken a cake decorating course and can make a birthday cake that rivals the ones we used to buy. Our new routines are well established and it's getting hard to remember life with gluten.

Because support groups have been so helpful to me, I have helped to form the Gluten-Free Group of Arizona, which offers support to the gluten-free and wheat-free community in Arizona. This includes adults, children, and their loved ones who avoid gluten due to celiac disease, gluten intolerance, dermatitis herpetiformis, autism, multiple sclerosis, rheumatoid arthritis and wheat allergies. We promote awareness of gluten-free issues, announce events in the gluten-free community and assist with member concerns and questions. As a chapter of the Gluten Intolerance Group, we also offer education through special events in our community and family-friendly support group meetings in the Phoenix/Chandler area of Arizona. (More information is available at www.glutenfreegroup.com.)

I'll admit there are many things that I still find hard. I'm a stay-at-home mom and I do a lot of volunteer work. Since being diagnosed, I generally avoid the luncheon meetings. These are mostly single menu events and I hate having to interrogate people about the food and then explain why I can't eat certain items. I'm hoping I'll get past this emotional hurdle in the near future.

Recently, we've had other health challenges arise in our family that put celiac disease into perspective. I have finally worked through my initial feelings (primarily anger and sadness) and am grateful that celiac disease is not cancer, lupus, or mental illness. It does not require painful medical treatments or medication with terrible side effects. It simply requires that we follow a gluten-free diet to be restored to health. On balance, that's not a bad deal. 🖎

Sue's son, Kevin, has written "Who Wants A Cookie?" which can be read in Chapter Four and her daughter, Angie, has written "My First Gluten-Free Halloween," which can be read later in this chapter.

Joy Of Celiac

by Jeanne Donnelly

I wrote this poem to express to the other celiacs I have met on the Internet how thankful I am for their help, encouragement and support. I don't know what I would have done without them!

The Doctor's voice was quiet
He gave a little shrug
"You have celiac sprue."
I asked, "Is that some kind of bug?"

"Oh no, just be careful."
He was kind of cheery now.
He handed me a list of food,
I could <u>not</u> eat, oh wow!

There's pizza on this list
And birthday cake here too!
And as I read it to the end
I never felt so blue.

To the Internet I ran
Fear clutching at my heart
To discover if there was a chance
That pasta and I would not part!

Then there on the net
A wondrous thing appeared
A whole celiac community
It wasn't as bad as I feared.

They taught me many things
How to shop and bake with care
This celiac thing got easier
Just because these folks were there.

So now I read the label
Of each can or jar or bottle
It's not really so bad
My tummy just needs to be coddled

But at least I have an answer
Though recovery may not be fast
All those years of suffering
Will soon be in the past!

Jeanne has also written "Confessions Of An Undiagnosed Celiac," which can be read in Chapter One.

Learning To Love Living With Celiac

by Cari Dorsey

I live with my husband, Jeff, and our three children, Shelby, Karsyn, and Brian in Augusta, Georgia. Jeff, Shelby, Karsyn, and I were all diagnosed with celiac disease in the spring of 2003.

We stumbled onto the diagnosis of celiac disease. For us, there wasn't a long, frustrating, exhausting search for an answer. We weren't looking for a new diagnosis for our 11-year-old daughter. Shelby had already been diagnosed one-and-a-half years earlier with reflex sympathetic dystrophy (RSD), a painful neuropathy disease affecting her left leg. She had also been experiencing severe chest pain for four months and we were concerned the RSD had moved into her chest. It was decided that an endoscopy might give us a clearer picture of what was going on inside. Biopsies were to be taken of her esophagus and stomach. It was unplanned, but our gastroenterologist also took biopsies from Shelby's small intestine.

The doctor called us with the results of Shelby's endoscopy. This was the first time we had ever heard of celiac disease. The biopsy showed there was villi damage in her intestines. Her subsequent lab work also proved positive. We scrambled to learn all we could about celiac disease. After searching three local bookstores, we could only find one book to get us started.

Our gastroenterologist had stressed the importance of beginning the diet immediately so we jumped into the diet with both feet. We spent hours on the Internet educating ourselves. We felt completely overwhelmed with trying to think of what we would be able to feed Shelby.

The feeling of being overwhelmed was soon replaced with excitement as the pain in Shelby's leg and chest lessened every day. Within two weeks we saw great improvement. RSD pain involves joints, bone aches, extreme sensitivity to touch and discoloration, to name only a few symptoms. These are also less common symptoms of celiac disease. While Shelby's diagnosis of RSD was correct, there is strong evidence that a gluten-free diet diminishes the RSD symptoms.

It was highly recommended by the gastroenterologist that the rest of the family be tested. Our youngest, Brian, now age seven, was diagnosed with dermatomyositis (DM), an autoimmune neuromuscular disease when he was three. We have learned research proves DM and celiac disease are related. We were relieved when our son's lab work and subsequent endoscopy came back negative for celiac.

Our daughter Karsyn's (age ten) test came back positive. Once we read the list of celiac symptoms, we knew that Karsyn would be positive. She had headaches, back pain, difficulty concentrating, and stomach aches to name a few of her common everyday complaints. We had taken her to see her pediatrician for all of these symptoms and they were each looked at individually. The pediatrician had different explanations for each of her symptoms.

To our surprise my husband Jeff's test and my test came back positive. We never dreamt we had celiac disease but amazingly, symptoms we had for years and had attributed to age and stress were greatly diminished within a week of going on a gluten-free diet. Our headaches, indigestion, chest pain, nausea, and extreme fatigue seemed to disappear.

We did not even realize how bad we were feeling on a day-to-day basis until our health improved.

Even though our son does not have celiac, we have eliminated all gluten from his diet since he does have an autoimmune disease linked with celiac. He needs very little encouragement to stay on the diet. He no longer complains of stomach pain or diarrhea.

We were certainly not experiencing what the medical doctors look for as typical celiac symptoms. None of us were losing weight or suffering from chronic diarrhea. We were not going from doctor to doctor looking for answers to serious health problems. If Shelby had not undergone an endoscopy, we would still be eating as we had before. We did not even realize how bad we were feeling on a day-to-day basis until our health improved.

We jumped immediately into the celiac diet. We completely re-organized the kitchen and eliminated any and all foods containing wheat and gluten. I went onto celiac Web sites and joined a few chat groups. We began compiling a three-ring binder of foods we could eat. I taught the girls how to call companies' 800 numbers and ask about the wheat and gluten status of their products, and then how to enter that information into our book. It wasn't long before life returned to "normal" at our house. Celiac is no longer the topic of all conversations but simply a way of life.

The girls are educated on the disease so they can eat out with friends and at their homes with confidence and without our help, as Brian will be when he is a little older. All of these things are important as it puts them in charge of the disease instead of the disease in charge of them.

We have been handed the key to a long life of good health. Every aspect of our lives has been affected.

In the short six months since Shelby was first diagnosed, our family had experienced many positive changes. While we weren't looking for celiac, we are grateful we were diagnosed in a timely manner.

There are seven celiacs in our extended family. We are able to be very supportive of each other. It is fun to try out gluten-free food together and to reminisce about foods we can no longer have. Our non-celiac family members are very cautious when they cook for us and take great care to only use appropriate ingredients and cooking methods. Almost all have educated themselves on the disease. They are now better able to understand our frustration, but what's more significant is they understand the importance of us strictly adhering to the diet and they encourage us to do so. They have witnessed the great improvements in our health.

We have been handed the key to a long life of good health. Every aspect of our lives has been affected. The children have handled it well and are grateful for the good health they are now experiencing. Several other members of our family have also been tested. I have a niece and a nephew who are also positive. When gluten is accidentally ingested, all of our symptoms vary greatly from one another. We don't worry about anyone "cheating" on the diet. The times we accidentally ingest gluten are enough to remind us how far we have come and we look forward to a healthy "gluten-free" life.

My First Gluten-Free Halloween

by Angie Clayton

I am six-years-old and live in Phoenix, Arizona. I'm in the first grade. I found out I had celiac disease the same week as my sixth birthday. My mother, father, and older brother all have celiac disease.

This was the first Halloween I couldn't eat any candy that had gluten in it. After we went trick or treating, I sorted my candy into a pile I could eat and a pile I could not eat. Then I decided to make a candy house, like a gingerbread house, out of the candy with gluten in it.

Mom made some icing and I spread it on a piece of cardboard. Then I unwrapped all my mini-chocolate bars to use as bricks. I used more icing as mortar to hold the bricks together. I built four walls doing this. I made a little roof using Kit Kat bars. On the walls without a roof, I decorated the top with gumdrops and other colorful candy. I stuck other candies in the mortar to make the house look pretty. I used icing around the house to make snow. I also used candy around the house to make pretty decorations in the snow. It was a beautiful house.

This was a lot more fun than having to throw away or give away my candy. I hope other kids will try this too. 🖎

Angie's older brother, Kevin, has written "Who Wants A Cookie," which can be read in Chapter Four and her mother, Sue, has written "Living With Celiac Disease: Our First Year," which can be read earlier in this chapter.

A Life Sentence, Not A Death Sentence

by Christina Kuhne

Celiac may be a life sentence but it is not a death sentence, and with knowledge and determination, I now know I can learn to live with it. To be told there was a name for what I have been suffering with for years and to be told I was not imagining it was the biggest relief I can remember.

Where Will I Begin?

I was diagnosed with celiac about five years ago. However, the problem began a long time before that. My life was dominated by frequent bouts of diarrhea and no way of knowing when they would hit. This led to many embarrassing moments and on a few occasions being "caught short."

My Most Embarrassing Moment

This was about a year before I was diagnosed. I was out shopping with my daughter and her friend and had to make a mad dash to the toilet, a common occurrence for me. Well we couldn't find one, and my daughter's friend was frantically trying to find one for me, but alas, it was too late. Without going into the details, I didn't make it and then had to sit in the public toilet while my daughter went and bought me some replacement clothes. I can still remember the feeling of disgust to this day.

If I can give anyone any advice, it is to learn as much as you can about the disease, the food you can eat, and the hidden sources of gluten in food.

How I Was Diagnosed

After several years my situation had developed to the stage where it seemed whatever I ate went straight through me. So I was back and forth to the doctors for all sorts of tests, which all came back negative. Since I was overweight, my doctor never thought of testing me for celiac disease. So let this be a warning, overweight people can have celiac.

One day I was moaning about my situation to a friend on the phone. As luck would have it she had another friend who had similar symptoms. She suggested I ring her friend who she said told her and I quote, "is on some special diet now and it works for her." So I rang and to my relief she knew exactly what I was talking about. She strongly suggested I return to my doctor and get tested for celiac.

With this information I trotted off to the doctor's office and she promptly ordered a blood test. The blood test indicated a positive result for celiac disease. Off to the specialist I went, who did all the tests and more. The final outcome: I indeed have celiac disease.

To my relief there was a name to this problem. I was not imagining it.

But I Had To Recover

The diet took a long time to learn because I thought like everyone else, "All right, no wheat, rye, barley, or oats." But there is a lot more to it than that. If I can give anyone any advice it is to learn as much as you can about the disease, the food you can eat, and the hidden sources of gluten in food. If possible, get rid of every product containing gluten in the house and if not keep your food very separate. As there is only my husband and me, I cook gluten-free and nothing else. My husband has his biscuits and bread but everything else is gluten-free.

Overcoming Other Problems

Because of the many years of living with the constant problem of diarrhea, and also due to the fact it had dominated my life for the past six months, I was left with panic attacks. They still affect me to this day and I don't think I will ever be free of the fear. But if you are suffering from panic attacks, let me tell you, you can conquer them. For me it was counseling and meditation. I had to teach my mind the difference between my imagined symptoms and the real symptoms. You will learn to tell the difference. I now know that in most cases an attack will occur usually within the hour and more than likely within three hours of ingesting something I shouldn't. I will get cramps and then diarrhea, but usually this lasts for about 30 minutes and then the fatigue sets in. If my symptoms are imagined as a result of panic then it is trip after trip to the toilet, usually not to do anything but to sit there and contemplate.

Where Will It End? With Hope

I could go on and on but this is just a brief extract of my experiences and I hope someone can learn something or get some comfort from them.

Celiac is a life sentence but not a death sentence. It is something we can learn to live with. Learn all you can, speak with all who have the knowledge. It takes time and effort but you, like me, can. There are thousands of others like us doing just that.

Good-Bye Letter To Gluten
by Rachel Smith

I noticed I was getting sick more often than not and decided to tell my doctor about it during my yearly check up. I didn't expect to find I had a disease called "Silly Yak!" I feel I have adjusted pretty well and go about my daily life continuing to do the things I love, such as playing the guitar, piano, singing, drawing, painting, reading, camping, hiking, and I even still enjoy cooking!

Dear Gluten,

What can I say? I've known you all of my life. You've been there when I was hungry and when I couldn't afford anything more than bread or ramen. I guess I didn't realize how important you have been to me, nor did I notice how many foods you are actually in! Thank you for all the times you were there for me but I have to say good-bye now.

You see, you are hurting me. I know you don't mean to but the reality is, you are. I can never eat you again. No more bread, pasta, or even canned soup. No more pizza at parties or a quick lunch with friends. I am sad to have to put you out of my life.

I have used you for many things, like socializing, comfort, and to fill my belly. Now I have to find different ways of doing that. I'm still not quite sure how to do it. I know part of why it is so difficult to just say good-bye and let go. I guess I've tried to just rely on myself to get through this farewell. I just can't do it alone. I have to rely on God. I know He is on my side and knows what a hardship this is for me.

Sometimes I am really confused at how much emotional connection and dependence I have had on you. I mean, you are just a "thing." I can live without you, love without you, and even eat without you. It's just that sometimes it doesn't feel like I can.

I still want to say good-bye. I know I can do it. I can be whole without you. I have God's help. I trust that I can and will get used to not having you around. I'll still miss you, but I don't need you. Other people can use you, that's okay. But me, I'll take the alternatives like a nice piece of rice bread! I know I will be better off without you.

Good-bye,
Rachel

Living With Celiac

Showing Real Intestinal Fortitude

> *Cake is something that I really miss,*
> *But my stomach keeps telling me this:*
> *If you don't eat the cake,*
> *There will be no tummy ache.*
> *A small price to pay for my bliss.*

One Molecule

by Ashley Reynolds-Rasmussen

I am a newlywed living in Columbia, Missouri. A recent college graduate, I enjoy going to flea markets, antique malls, and working with children.

I would like to dedicate this article to my grandmother, Jean Henry, who I've always had a special connection with. I would also like to thank everyone who has embraced me during years of struggling with my health. You have all touched my heart and will never be forgotten.

Before I start giving you advice and sharing my story, I should tell you a little about myself. My name is Ashley Reynolds-Rasmussen and I am 22 years old. I have been struggling with digestive problems for almost 15 years dealing with a very wide range of symptoms; everything from heartburn to diarrhea and severe vomiting which forced me to be put on a feeding tube. I have been through the entire collection of testing that is out there for digestive problems. Some of them multiple times. Over the course of all this testing, I have been diagnosed with no less than 15 diseases and conditions. However, I did not get a correct diagnosis of celiac disease until June 2002, by a doctor at the Mayo Clinic. I feel I have experienced much more in my 22 years of life than most people have in 80.

The most simplistic piece of advice I have received since being diagnosed with celiac disease is also what I now think is most important for newly diagnosed celiacs to hear. One molecule of gluten is the same as 10,000.

Each of us has our struggles. Some of us struggle with our weight, some of us struggle with money, and some of us struggle with back problems. What millions struggle with, but yet never seem to talk about, are digestive problems. Words such as diarrhea and stomach cramps are almost taboo in thousands of homes across America. With that being said, millions of people are suffering in silence and have nowhere to turn. Those of us who suffer from digestive problems whether it be weekly, monthly or daily, need to learn to speak out about our problems, and bring awareness to them. Awareness is what has scientists working on a cure for cancer and it is what will someday bring a cure to those of us suffering from celiac disease and other digestive problems.

The most simplistic piece of advice I have received since being diagnosed with celiac disease is also what I now think is most important for newly diagnosed celiacs to hear. One molecule of gluten is the same as 10,000 molecules. Take this statement as literally as it sounds. I have had experiences where my meal at a restaurant is completely gluten-free except for the bread that comes with it. I have learned the hard way you cannot simply take the bread off your plate when your order arrives. You must specifically order your meal with no bread. The bread must never touch your plate. If it does, you can have experiences like I have had, where you are sick by the time you leave the restaurant. This can get hard at restaurants where they think you just don't like bread. You must be strong and strict with your words and make it clear to them that no bread can touch your plate.

To take this piece of advice even further, something as small as stirring pasta with one spoon and then stirring gluten-free pasta with the same spoon, can make you sick. Treat gluten like it is, a deadly poison, and do all you can to not ingest any of it. Even if you are unable to see any gluten, it could be there. One molecule is very small!

The people you surround yourself with are an essential part of your recovery and your success in dealing and living with this disease. I have been very blessed with my new husband. Bryan rarely eats foods containing gluten around me. He is more than willing to try new gluten-free foods with me and to help me cook them. He accepts the fact I am not able to eat out anywhere we want and food is something I have to be constantly aware of. He is very aware that one molecule of gluten is the same as 10,000 and he never lets me forget it. All of this has been a huge help and part of my success in staying gluten-free.

Every celiac deserves a spouse or parent just like Bryan to support them and love them. There are people in my life that will still invite me to an all gluten containing meal and who are not willing to understand the impact gluten has on my health. These people are not respectful of me and therefore, not healthy for my recovery. People like Bryan are a very healthy part of my recovery.

Something else that has taken me almost 15 years to understand and believe is having a digestive disease like celiac is no different than being in a wheelchair or having some other condition that requires accommodations to be made. If someone in your family is in a wheelchair, you wouldn't take them to a non-handicapped accessible restaurant to eat. The same can be said about someone with celiac disease. Even though I spread the word to my friends and family about celiac disease and exactly what it is, some family members still invited me to eat out at an Italian restaurant. I went along, not having the courage to speak up for myself and sat through dinner with an empty plate. In retrospect, I should have never put myself in that situation. I should have spoken up and requested we go to a different restaurant where it would have been easier for me to find something to eat. Wheelchair bound people would never say "yes" to a restaurant they cannot get into and so why should we?

Finally, there are people who say we should not let this disease control our lives. I used to believe that, but now I believe we should. We must follow its strict rules and by following those rules we can finally start to feel normal again. We should change our lives and habits to make them gluten-free. We must also remember the positive impact this disease has made upon our lives. It is easy for us to only remember the negatives when smelling freshly cooked cinnamon rolls or driving past a fast food restaurant. This disease has helped to make me who I am today and I am proud of that person.

Ashley's mother, Marilyn Carr, has written "I'll Make A Deal With You God," which can be read in Chapter Five.

How Belly Dancing Saved My Life

by Carman Theis

Mild mannered computer programmer by day, international dancer by night. I work full time developing database programs for the Internet. I also have two side businesses, one as a professional belly dancer, one as an importer and reseller of accessories for the dance community. It is frightening to know that even at its worst, my illness went completely unnoticed to those who were the closest in my life. I was completely on my own until very recently, with no one to help me with the day to day issues, except for the growing celiac community on the Internet. Fortunately through my dance I found the self-awareness, strength and persistence to recognize something was seriously wrong, then to find the solution, and finally to make the necessary dramatic life changes necessary for recovery. I would not be alive today if it were not for my dance.

You never know how sick you are until you start to get better. That pretty much sums up my whole story. Three years ago I made my first trip to Cairo for two weeks of shopping, dancing, and mingling with the local culture. It was an extraordinary trip, made all the more exciting by the fact my friend and I traveled on our own without the benefit of a tour group or guide. It was not until our last day that I fell prey to the usual traveler's sickness. On my return, I did the usual thing. I waited a few days for it to subside, and then I made an appointment with my doctors. I was given a course of antibiotics and told not to worry, "It will go away in time." But it never did.

Then I learned about gluten intolerance and celiac disease. I tried to discuss the idea I might be gluten intolerant with my doctor, but he said it was not possible because I was not losing weight.

Meanwhile, I started getting compliments on my new relaxed, naturally languid style of dancing that was very "Egyptian." It was very different from my previously very energetic Turkish-inspired style. I thought it was because I learned how to feel the music more. The real issue was I physically had less energy, and didn't notice it. All I knew is I often felt so depressed for no apparent reason that even waking up in the morning was an effort. I literally lived day-to-day. I didn't care to make goals for the future.

Still my stomach issues persisted. I patiently waited for them to resolve. Finally, I had an epiphany moment. An SUV almost ran me off the road on Christmas Eve. My car was totaled, but I walked away with only a bump on my wrist. I realized I had to take care of myself because no one else would.

Thus began a journey that changed my life in ways I would never have imagined. I returned to my doctors to take care of my health issues. Two years earlier I had been diagnosed with rosacea, a skin condition that was causing progressive damage to the skin on my face that could not be hidden by make-up. This was hard to deal with as I believed I may never be able to realize my dreams as a performer.

I was determined to not let this stop me and started doing some research. I learned a change in diet could reverse this condition and control it enough that I could stop the daily medications. I was ecstatic. The diet was very restrictive. You start by eating no more than 20 grams of carbohydrates a day for the first 30 days, then work to find your tolerance level. No sugars in any form. No bread or pasta. No more spicy food. No hot or cold food or beverages. I needed to avoid anything that caused my face to blush after eating it. Add to that behavior changes such as: avoiding hot showers, sun, outdoor exposure, and exercise. But I was determined. I wanted to continue performing! I returned to my dermatologist and shared my research with her. She felt it was worth a try!

I also returned to my primary care physician regarding my lingering stomach issues. We did test after test after test with no solution. I was convinced I had picked up a bug in Cairo. But then something amazing happened. A month after I changed to my rosacea diet, my stomach issues started

At my last appointment with the doctor, he handed down a diagnosis of irritable bowel syndrome. Many times this is a diagnosis given when a doctor can't figure out what is wrong, as in my case.

to resolve. I shared this information with my doctor, and he encouraged me to eat whatever way made me feel better. He assured me that the changes in my diet would not affect his tests.

As time went on, I researched to learn why my diet was affecting my stomach so much. I tried a low glycemic diet. Still I had periodic issues. Then I learned about gluten intolerance and celiac disease. I tried to discuss the idea I might be gluten intolerant with my doctor, but he said it was not possible because I was not losing weight. He also said he did that test as a part of the first round of tests. He hinted the dietary affect could be all in my head, and gave me a sample pack of Metamucil to try.

I wasn't convinced my doctor was right, so I made a point of getting a copy of the tests and I checked the hospital records myself. I was very angry to see he did not do the correct tests. The celiac blood test panel consists of four tests. He only did one, the one which tests for short term (recent) exposure to gluten. Plus, the hospital record said right on the test description, a change in diet to exclude gluten will affect the results.

I was livid. At the time of the test I had been off all obvious forms of gluten (bread, pasta, cookies, cakes, etc.) for at least a month. I was already feeling improvement on the diet because my body was healing. By the time I saw the hospital record, I had been off gluten for several months. Yet, he had reassured me on three separate occasions a change in diet would not affect the test results. Add to that his offhand comment that it was all in my head. He was trying to treat me for a condition he knew nothing about, pretending he knew what he was doing. I discovered the Internet celiac community, and learned a great deal. However the doctor dismissed any information I found through my research when I brought it up for discussion.

Time went on as I endured medical test after test. I

quickly learned I had to take charge of my own case. Suddenly at month five I woke up. I felt better. I had a brain! I could actually work a full day without a nap in the middle. I could think clearly, as if someone had swept all the cobwebs out of my brain. I could focus on complicated things. I started to dream of the future.

At my last appointment with the doctor, he handed down a diagnosis of irritable bowel syndrome. Many times this is a diagnosis given when a doctor can't figure out what is wrong, as in my case. I insisted on a referral to a gastrointestinal specialist, and he promptly gave me one. My new doctor was almost as dismissive (at that time celiac was thought to be extremely rare in the United States, at less than 1 in 3000). I was almost in tears as I told him my case had been mishandled from the start. He started asking questions about my observations and my family history. He concluded that indeed I seemed to be at least gluten sensitive, and ordered all the correct tests to find out. At our next appointment I reminded him, even as I was going under sedation for the endoscopy, that I had been off gluten for at least eight months and experienced many signs of recovery. It was unlikely he would find any obvious damage to my system. As expected, the endoscopy and all four blood tests came up negative. But the gastroenterologist maintained I was obviously gluten sensitive and should remain on a gluten-free diet.

But something was not quite right. I still reacted periodically to foods manufactured specifically to be gluten-free. I went to see an allergist to figure out why. My skin prick tests came up negative. I was advised to keep a food diary and try an elimination diet to identify the offending foods.

So I started my rotation elimination diet. This is a very difficult task that most fail, but I was determined. I learned over time I could not tolerate dairy, soy or eggs. I've also learned it is common for celiacs to have additional food reactions as a direct result of the damage to their system. Some reactions may go away with time, and some may be an issue forever. My allergist was so impressed with my rotation elimination diet and food diary system, she asked for a copy to use as an example for other patients. She later asked for my restaurant cards as well.

I woke up one morning realizing for the first time in my life my tummy was becoming flat. This was amazing. I thought I would live life always having to accommodate a rounded bulging lower belly in my costume designs. I even once considered cosmetic surgery to correct it. And here it was almost gone! I've even noticed dramatic differences in my energy and flexibility when I am clear of food reactions. My dermatologist (remember her?) remarked my facial skin was improving so much that I should continue whatever I was doing. My medication dosage was dropped twice. If I continue to improve, perhaps one day I will be able to stop the medications entirely. It was amazing that a "simple" change in diet could improve so many seemingly unrelated things. I felt reborn. I was excited to be alive. I felt like I had a second chance to achieve my dreams.

The changes have been profound. I can no longer eat in restaurants without anxiety. I can no longer trust others to prepare foods for me. I need to be careful to always wash my hands before touching food I plan to eat. I can't lick stamps and envelopes. I had to replace all of the spices in my kitchen, as well as most of the food and several pans and cooking utensils. I had to learn to read ingredients not only in foods, but also medications, cosmetics and household products. I had to learn not to trust ingredient lists because they are often incomplete. I have to be very careful around children. I have to be very careful not to eat anything risky for at least four days before a performance. Every time I eat, do makeup, or pay bills, it is an opportunity to poison myself. A single molecule of contamination can make me ill for a week. Continued contamination can even kill me.

But life is good. I am working with a new personal trainer to regain the strength and endurance I lost in my illness, as well as develop muscle tone in places I never dreamed possible. For once in my life, I can have that perfect body, the body perfect for me. I never could have done it if it weren't for my dancing. Something about having to look gorgeous in a revealing costume, drag myself out the door, bring happiness to others and dance my cares away on a regular basis made it so much more crucial to persist at finding the solution to my health issues. Something about having to do this every single weekend made it possible to follow my new diet long enough to heal and realize the benefits of these restrictions for their own merits.

If it weren't for my belly dancing, I would probably not be alive today. And for once in my life, I am truly alive. ✍

Be Positive

by Sharla Wiatt

I am a 31-year-old second grade teacher. I discovered I had problems with gluten when I was getting sinus infections monthly and had severe allergies. It wasn't until I realized that my mom's rash was DH and my four-year-old daughter was having reoccurring tummy aches that I went gluten-free. My allergies are now gone and I haven't had a sinus infection since.

When my doctor first told me I needed to stop eating gluten I thought he was crazy. What was I supposed to eat if I couldn't have any bread? I decided since I was only suffering from allergies and sinus headaches I would try my best to stay away from any gluten, but it wouldn't hurt if I had just a little bit.

It wasn't until my four-year-old daughter started having tummy aches that I decided I better get a little more serious about being gluten-free. I thought if my daughter has to eat this way then I should do the same.

Amazingly, after about a month of being off gluten, all of my allergies seemed to go away. I was no longer taking Allegra-D every day along with Sudafed, and a nasal spray. My headaches also seemed to decrease as well. I did begin to develop some other food allergies as my body was healing. Since I started rotating the foods I have trouble with I rarely have headaches anymore.

At first a gluten-free diet is very tough and it seems like it will never get easy, however it does. I have found that having a positive attitude has helped tremendously. Instead of thinking of all of the foods I can't have, I think of all of the wonderful foods I can have. I have learned to bake (which I never thought possible). Since I've been on the diet I am not so tired all of the time. I find I have more energy and I use it to bake breads, cakes and cookies for my family. I am beginning to realize there aren't too many foods that can't be transformed into gluten-free.

My daughter doesn't seem to feel left out because I am always prepared. I am in the habit of bringing snacks with us wherever we go. Trail mixes, gluten-free pretzels, protein bars, and fruit are easy to take, just in case. I also freeze cupcakes or brownies to bring along with us to birthday parties. We don't make a big deal about it, therefore other people don't make a big deal.

We also joined a wonderful support group in our area. Just talking with other people that have the same problem helps tremendously. We have ordered gluten-free products together which saves money on the shipping and handling. We also share our favorite products and recipes. One member of our group even organized a gluten-free pizza party at a pizza parlor!

I guess I am just thankful that my daughter and I are healthy and happy. What other disease can you have that is so easy to fix?

Repair Work
(or Knit One, Purl Two)
by Christie Schroeter

I worked as a reporter for the Austin American-Statesman newspaper in Austin, Texas, for 13 years. I am now a freelancer and writing for various publications. In 1995 my health took a downward plunge. All the classic celiac symptoms manifested themselves, but doctors did not diagnose the disease for two-and-a-half years. In that time, I became unable to work and barely able to cope with the simplest of household tasks. After finding a gastroenterologist who correctly diagnosed the problem, I became a strong advocate of reaching out to others who share this disease. My writing on this subject is one way I accomplish this goal.

My grandmother laughed as she watched me struggle to learn how to knit. She had tried to teach me, but maybe it wasn't just a lack of coordination on my part. Possibly it was more a lack of wanting to learn. Nana gently took the knitting needles from me as we sat side-by-side on the couch, and began to try and fix my work. I enjoyed watching her deft movements, ones she could do in her sleep from all the practice she had in this craft.

My thoughts drift back to that moment when I think about the repair work my body has been doing since I went on a gluten-free diet six years ago. I can't see it taking place, but remarkable changes in my health and energy level are proof-positive that it's happening. It didn't take place overnight, however. In fact, it was such a slow process that in the beginning I doubted I would ever regain the "old me."

Immediately after discovering I had celiac disease, I eliminated all gluten sources from my diet. The worst of the symptoms I had been experiencing for over two years disappeared quite rapidly, which was encouraging, to say the least. But then, what I like to refer to as "bouts of gluten-like attacks" came and went on a fairly regular basis. I was also still extremely fatigued. When would I heal?

Since I've never been a shy one about asking for help, I immediately contacted the Gluten Intolerance Group of North America (GIG). A feeling of relief came over me as I talked with one of their volunteers who advised me not to become anxious. Healing takes time, she said, adding that it's a day-to-day process. The damage done over a period of years would take time to fix. That calm advice led me to my next plan of action, which was to get in touch with my local celiac support group.

What a wealth of information I gleaned from these knowledgeable members. One kind lady actually took me shopping at a natural food store so we could go aisle by aisle and read labels together. I learned about how many hidden sources of gluten are lurking in the most innocent looking foods. I became savvy in knowing what to buy and what to avoid. Bit by bit the puzzle came together. I discovered that lactose intolerance is very common in people with newly diagnosed celiac disease. From that, milk and all milk products were eliminated from my personal food pyramid, producing quick results in doing away with the bowel problems.

Other food allergies, once uncovered, were instrumental in continuing the healing process. Soy, another big allergen for many folks, was checked off my list, too. Every time I would eat a cracker or piece of gluten-free bread containing soy, my body would respond with negative results. I had to literally start with one basic food, which in my case was rice, and then add another to test the waters.

Looking back, I realize my repair work has been ongoing. Family members have commented over and over how much healthier I look. Foods I was unable to digest a few years ago are now ones I can enjoy. I still recall the first time I was able to sit down to a heaping portion of broccoli and eat it to my heart's content. A bowl of pinto beans.....unheard of at our house for many moons due to my wimpy digestive tract, is now a frequent dish. I cannot claim lactose intolerance anymore, to my great relief. Bring on the difficult to digest foods! I'm ready for them. My knitting and purling has finally become an art form in this body of mine. ✍

It Gets Better

by Jenn Cain

I am a community and school advocate for prevention of youth use of drugs and alcohol. I work with schools, youth, police, parents and local governments to make sure kids are supported in such a way that they make better choices and become productive and successful citizens.

I won't go into the gory details of how long I was sick and how I found out I had celiac. I will say I was anemic, and after months of non-responsive iron consumption, my general doctor suspected an "absorption problem." A visit to the gastroenterologist and the rest is history.

On one hand I was relieved to find an answer but on the other hand, it slowly became clear to me I was clueless as to what was really involved in recovery. What I did know was I had to be careful and once diagnosed, I NEVER purposefully ingested gluten. However, it was my children that recognized the danger of using the family butter tub, jelly, peanut butter, etc. It was my ever-vigilant daughter who would yell at others to be careful when my eyes couldn't be everywhere. It was the local celiac group, the Internet, some lessons in assertiveness and reading, reading labels that would teach me how to be safe. I knew it would take time, patience, and dedication to become healthy and the thought of good health is what got me through.

But something was bothering me. I was having mood swings and at times I wasn't very pleasant. I didn't even know how I'd feel from one moment to the next. I thought I was being jealous, or maybe a little self-pitying when I would walk between the vendors at a country fair and become cognizant there was nothing I could safely eat (I miss tempura). I thought it was unfair when my colleagues would bring éclairs to work and speak so lovingly of their flavor and texture. I really started to get pissed off when my family continued their tradition of pizza night and left me to fend for myself.

Then I realized I was grieving. I had lost something that was wonderful; the ability to enjoy any food I wanted any time I wanted. I've worked with amputees and spinal cord injuries, how could I be grieving about something as trivial as not being able to eat a donut? But it doesn't matter. Grief is grief, and loss is loss and shouldn't be compared. Once I understood what I was going through, it helped me cope. I stopped saying "I can't" when offered food by my fellow wheat-eaters and started saying "no, thank you." (Although I often advocate for celiac awareness, I can tell when people aren't interested.) I started sharing stories of the wonderful food I was enjoying like homemade stir-fry, crust-less pumpkin pie with whipped cream and crumbled gluten-free ginger snaps, rice noodle lasagna (that my non-celiac family preferred), and many other creative and delicious concoctions.

It's been over five years now, and the moments of regret get fewer and fewer while the moments of excitement increase. Every trip to the grocery store, I find more and more promising food items. I've found it helpful to bring my cell phone with me so I can call manufacturers from the store. I've discovered Snapple makes a delicious meal replacer drink, Progresso makes a creamy mushroom soup that rivals any memory of Cambells, and joy of joys, there is a gluten-free beer on the horizon. I recently visited Whole Foods and found that Amy's is making a rice crust frozen pizza. I ran to the car and called my mother who lived nearby and told her to preheat her oven because I was stopping by to cook a pizza (I didn't want to wait the 45 minutes till I got home).

So for you newbies, it will get easier and better and life will become fun again. It's okay to be sad. It's okay to be mad. It's part of the process of accepting the incredible limitations associated with celiac. It can also be part of growing to become a more compassionate and understanding human being. Oh yeah, and one more thing, I really, REALLY love Edy's peppermint ice cream with a little Hershey's chocolate sauce.

Grief

by R. Jean Powell

*In 1991 I was formally diagnosed with celiac disease and
began my dedicated work with Montana Celiac patients. In
collaboration with Lily Patten and Eloise Faber, Montana Celiac
Society was born, with a founding membership of seven. The
quarterly newsletter, Gluten-Free Friends, was founded in 1994
when I became editor. Circulation today is 620 and growing. This
number includes over 550 subscribing families and nearly 50
clinics, hospitals and medical personnel in Montana who receive
complimentary issues as part of our drive to educate.*

My mother was the classic chronic celiac, not
diagnosed until two years before her death at
83, when I was diagnosed. The ancestral trail
led to an Irish great grandmother who died in her late forties
of "stomach trouble." There were four siblings in my mom's
family, and in retrospect we know that only my Aunt Addie
escaped the celiac genes. My grandfather was the legendary
"skipped generation."

I have two daughters, a daughter-in-law, and a grandchild
who have celiac disease. I also have one son who, at forty,
remains alert to the possibility of inheriting the gene.

I am a native Montanan who was diagnosed in 1981 with

multiple sclerosis. In the next 10 years, I became gradually more ill with puzzling symptoms unrelated to my multiple sclerosis. Bedridden by 1990, I developed severe diarrhea. Researching the causes of the many symptoms I was experiencing, I was led again and again to celiac disease and was referred to a skeptical gastroenterologist. Displaying typical crisis symptoms, showing an immediate response to the diet, and with a generations-long genetic history of comparable family health problems, I was formally diagnosed with celiac disease. I am healthy today, but was left with a permanent walking disability.

Grief is a normal reaction to losses in one's life, but the power of normal grief can be overlooked by family, friends, even physicians after patients receive a specific diagnosis of celiac disease.

If you were fortunate to have been given the diagnosis of celiac disease then eventually you will come to terms with your topsy-turvy new universe and life-style. But first you must deal with your bereavement. You are not the person you thought you were, and you grieve for your lost self. You've lost years of good health, opportunities, and peace of mind. Your family history may include pointless tragedies and unnecessary early deaths. You flounder with feelings of anger, even rage, which prevent a sense of well-being. To top it off, you wonder how you can survive without bread, the staff of life. You're scared…

If you had been very ill, perhaps for years, the relief at feeling better will soften the edges of your anguish, but grieving is a process each diagnosed celiac person must experience. As we wend our individual ways through the normal stages of grief that range from shock, anger, denial, numbness, sadness, to a final appreciative acceptance, we need reassurance that one day soon we will approach our special, and peculiar, circumstances with gratitude.

This journey can take as long as two years, but should grief remain unacknowledged, it can turn into habitual depression. So be kind and loving to your own sadness or it may sneak up and bite you with unexpected small sorrows throughout your life.

Cherish the reality: no surgery, no expensive medication, no chemical therapy, but the avoidance of wheat, rye, and barley is the treatment prescribed. With conscientious management, your health will rebound. It is your second chance to live optimistically, expressing hope and gratitude while enjoying the multitude of blessings that include a very good diet, gluten-free!

R. Jean Powell is the author of a children's book "A Sweet Fairy Tale©, A Satire." It is spiral bound, in color with graphics. Its advanced text makes it perfect for readers ten and older but younger children will enjoy the colorful and fun graphics as the book is read to them.

The book is designed to help children develop a good attitude toward the gluten-free diet using a familiar children's format, the fairy tale. Characters include: Ricerella, Tiny Crumb, Gliadin the bad witch and her cat, Blacktoes, and others.

If you wish to order the book send $12.50 + $2.00 postage per copy in check or money order to:

R. Jean Powell
1019 South Bozeman Avenue, #3
Bozeman, Montana 59715
(406) 586-1285

Gluten Paranoia?
(or, How I Stopped Defining Myself By My Disease)

by Marge Johannemann

I am a retired nurse who lives with my husband of 41 years, Bill. We have three sons who each have two sons for a total of six grandsons. They range in age from 3 to 18 years old. Two of our grandsons are intolerant to gluten, casein, and yeast. This was determined through Dr. Kenneth Fine's Enterolab. Their father is also intolerant to gluten.

I was diagnosed with celiac disease in July of 1994 and held the first meeting of the Greater Louisville Celiac Sprue Support Group in March of 1995. I served as founder, president, and newsletter editor for two years. I now serve as contributing editor and education advisor. My hobbies are long distance bicycling, gardening, and reading.

Answer the following questions:

1-Do you avoid going out to restaurants because you are afraid you will be exposed to gluten?

2-Do you shy away from family gatherings because you don't think there will be anything for you to eat?

3-Are you constantly calling food manufacturers to determine if gluten is in a product even though the label does not indicate gluten is present?

4-Do you avoid many foods fearing there may be cross-contamination?

5-Have you limited yourself to a minimal variety of foods because you are afraid of coming in contact with gluten?

6-Do you find yourself hungry or unsatisfied after eating only those foods you are sure do not contain gluten?

7-Are you constantly expressing fears you may have about ingesting gluten?

8-Do you now define yourself as a celiac?

If you are new to the gluten-free diet, this is the natural part of becoming accustomed to a new lifestyle that limits foods containing wheat, rye, barley, and oats. There is definitely a huge learning curve when it comes to reading labels and understanding the ingredients contained therein. It does take time to learn the vocabulary of ingredients derived from the offending grains. There is also some time needed to grieve for the loss of your old gluten-containing lifestyle. After all, things were much easier before the diagnosis of celiac disease or gluten intolerance, and you may have spent years getting the proper diagnosis.

It occurred to me I am not a celiac. I am a person who happens to be intolerant to gluten. Once my gut was healed, I no longer suffered from a disease.

I remember well my reaction to the diagnosis. I was grateful I wasn't imagining my symptoms. I could actually put a name on my ailment. I felt validated. I didn't have cancer. I could get better. All I had to do was stay away from gluten!

As I traveled my road to recovery, not knowing another living person with my problem and not having access to the Web, I began to find out that living my life gluten-free, while it made me feel better, was no piece of cake (gluten-free, of course)!

I had to learn to cook in a different way. Suddenly I was saddled with the task of making bread; something I had never done. And this bread contained ingredients I had never heard of much less used. I was cooking more than I had ever cooked before. This was just at the time when our last child had left home and my husband and I were enjoying the freedom of eating out whenever we wished.

It definitely put a cramp in my social life. For a long time, I felt I would never again be spontaneous. Everywhere I went I took food with me, fearing there would be nothing gluten-free available to eat. I found myself staying at home more because of the diet restrictions. For a long while, my entire life evolved around obtaining and creating gluten-free food. How lucky I was to have the support of my husband and family during this time. I couldn't have done it without them.

Probably the best thing that came out of my struggle (and anger) was founding our support group. I was determined that other people would never have to adopt this lifestyle alone. I literally spent the next five or so years with a daily focus on spreading the word about celiac disease. Talking with newly diagnosed celiacs, assisting undiagnosed celiacs in getting a proper diagnosis, educating doctors, training dietitians, attending national conferences and meetings, writing articles for publication, and getting the word out in every way I could.

You know what? One day I realized there is more to life than celiac disease. While I have never regretted doing all the things I did, I began to realize there are other important things I had neglected for a long time. What about my overall health? My family and friends? My need to be creative in other ways? The importance of just taking a day off to read, to visit with friends, to garden, to ride my bicycle or to do nothing at all?

It occurred to me I am not a celiac. I am a person who happens to be intolerant to gluten. Once my gut was healed, I no longer suffered from a disease. This breakthrough made me see myself, once again, as me - the total person!

No longer do I obsess over gluten. I just do my best within reason to remain gluten-free. I very seldom call a food company about ingredients, partly because I have a better knowledge of those ingredient words we all have to learn. But mostly, because I read the label and if I don't see anything to be alarmed about, I go ahead and use the product. So far, I am doing very well health-wise. As a matter of fact, I am healthier now than I have ever been. Probably because I use my time to exercise, eat properly, and get plenty of rest and relaxation.

I don't even call pharmaceutical companies any more unless a medication is prescribed for me for long term use. I don't get concerned about things like antibiotics, pain medication, and other short-term prescriptions. I have finally realized there are sometimes worse health problems than celiac disease. And if the doctor prescribes a particular medication to assist me in the short term, then it is probably wise for me to take it.

I have a much more active social life now that I have stopped defining myself as a celiac. I don't even talk about it with others very often. After all, who wants to hear about my intestinal problems? My friends already know I can't just eat anything I want and they are very supportive by asking me what ingredients to use when they are going to cook for me.

I again love to eat out. Depending on where I will be eating, I usually don't call about ingredients. Instead, I ask how they prepare their food after I get there. I might say I can't eat wheat and if they assume it's because of an allergy, I just let them think that. I guess I'm just tired of going through the whole explanation. I usually do pretty well with my new approach. Occasionally, I do have to send something back to the kitchen, but it really doesn't happen that often.

I am always courteous when asking about food preparation, but I also let the server or chef know the importance of having my food the way I would like it. You don't have to be belligerent or unkind about this. You can be firm and nice and still get what you need. So far, this has worked very well for me. Much better than using one of the well-touted restaurant cards that usually only scare the server or chef into believing they cannot feed me at all.

At this point in my life I have already lived the greater part of it, and I don't care to sweat the small stuff. I live a very full life and I have many friends and interests. The last thing I care to worry about is gluten! Not to say I don't pay attention, but I do my very best to remain gluten-free while enjoying my life to the fullest. If I occasionally, unknowingly get some gluten, I refuse to obsess about it. Life is short and I plan to live it to the fullest!

A Trip To The Hospital
by Mary Minnich

I am currently a stay-at-home mom, though I worked as a nurse for many years. I home school my three celiac children, while my adopted son attends the local high school. We live on a small farm and raise donkeys, goats, and chickens. I've been cooking gluten-free since my husband discovered he had celiac disease ten years ago. Three years ago, I discovered I too was sensitive to gluten.

My greatest challenge with celiac disease occurred when my nine-year-old son, Michael, required hospitalization. Michael asked if he could go play at a friend's house. I agreed and a little while later I was surprised when his friend showed up at my door beckoning me to come quickly. Michael was hurt and his friend's mom had called for an ambulance.

I grabbed my shoes and cell phone and hurried over the chairs the boys used to get across the fence in our adjoining backyards. I arrived at the neighbor's house to see my son lying on a carpet with a blood soaked towel pressed to his chest and abdomen. I am a nurse, but nothing quite prepared me for seeing my child in that condition.

My friend filled me in on what happened. Michael had

been climbing a tree and the branch broke. As he fell, he got caught on another branch, which penetrated his skin. She had lifted him out of the tree and carried him into the house.

The ambulance arrived and they worked to stabilize him for transport. They asked me for a medical history and I told them asthma, no drug allergies, but he does have celiac. I vaguely remember giving them details of what celiac was, recalling that I knew little about it before members of my family were diagnosed. As they loaded Michael into the ambulance, they told me to meet them at the nearest hospital. I had been trying to locate my husband at work, but was only able to leave a message on the voice mail. As I hurried home to get my van for the trip to the hospital, I called a friend, telling her I was scared Michael would not make it. I received a call, the paramedics had changed their minds and were taking him to the trauma center at another hospital.

I drove to the hospital and was told Michael needed emergency surgery. The surgery went well, but Michael was going to need to stay in the hospital a week for antibiotics.

After the shock of the experience wore off a bit, we started dealing with the necessity of finding food for a celiac boy with a lot of tissue to heal. As I expected, the nursing staff didn't have much knowledge of the condition. It wasn't something I remembered studying in nursing school. I asked to speak to the dietician and we spent some time going over menus. It turned out the special children's menu items were all full of gluten. The dietician did her best to come up with some alternatives, but the selection was very limited.

We finally got an okay for a hot dog, no bun for lunch that day. Lunchtime came, and so did his tray. I lifted the cover to find the hot dog, but right next to it was a slice of white bread. I had to laugh. It was then I realized the hospital was no place for someone with celiac. Michael got tired of the same options on the menu so when he was able to leave the unit, the dietician gave him a meal ticket to pick out his own food in the cafeteria. We went through the line: breaded meat, meat soaked in gravy and pasta dishes. Unfortunately the salad bar was closed at dinnertime. We got Michael a large juice from the beverage cooler, and headed for the gift shop to see if we could find something there. Their main item was sandwiches. No help there. That's when we discovered a certain kind of ice-cream bar was gluten-free. It became a once a day ritual during the rest of his stay.

It occurred to me to make a trip to the grocery store, but every time I mentioned leaving for an errand, my son's eyes would water and his lip would quiver, so I stayed. My friends were calling to check on us. They'd ask, "What can I do?" The answer was always "Bring food!" You see, I was having an even harder time finding something for me to eat since I didn't have a dietician working for me. One friend was very educated about the celiac diet and went to the grocery for us. She came in carrying several bags of groceries and loaded them into the closet. She also brought some food from one of my favorite restaurants. What a change from ice-cream bars, candy and chips. With the help of the dietician and my friends, Michael and I survived that week in the hospital, but it was so good to return home and back to my gluten-free kitchen. Cooking dinner never felt so good. 🖋

My Hospital Story

by Erica Wilson

I am a 46-year-old Floridian who is a transplant from Pennsylvania. I am the mother of three children, one married, one in college, and one living at home. After years of frustration, I discovered I was a celiac at the age of 27. This story is about my first hospital experience.

One would think a hospital, of all places, would be able to handle a special diet, especially a hospital in a large city like Miami. It was a "Catch 22" for me. They bring you all your meals so you must depend on them to be correct and not make you sicker than when you went into the hospital. You can't easily go down to the cafeteria or whip up a meal on a hot plate. As it turned out, my ailment was almost the easiest part of my stay.

After talking to other celiacs, I thought I wouldn't have to live their horror stories if I talked to the dietitian a day before my planned stay. That is precisely what I did when I went in for some blood tests two days before I was admitted. The dietician was a young girl probably not out of school for more than six months to a year. She seemed sympathetic to my gluten-free plea but kept telling me about how short they were in kitchen staff.

I just couldn't imagine what it would have been like if I hadn't spoken to the dietitian. My first gourmet course was something that resembled chicken soup (the French chef must have been off that day). Included with the soup were three juicy cellophane wrapped saltine crackers. Needless to say, all I ate was the red apple. Luckily for me I didn't feel like eating much anyway.

My husband is a super guy and brought me a care package of snacks. The next day I was on IV and they couldn't mess that up too badly. By day three I was feeling better and decided to make it my mission to teach the nurses about celiac disease. Much to my surprise they were clueless, but eager to listen to my plea.

My best advice for myself, and anyone else who has to do the hospital thing, would be to get a doctor involved. Hopefully his orders would be followed better than our requests. I would also pack a lunch or two. I know what is in what I make. Don't assume the hospital is going to get it right. Do everything you can so your stay doesn't make you any sicker.

I Miss Oreo Biscuits

by *Amelia Dani*

I am six years old and I live with my mum, dad, brother, and sister. I was very small for my age but I have now caught up and my skin problems have cleared up because of my new diet. I love swimming, my pet cat, Shadow, and being with my friends. Having celiac disease has not held me back.

My name is Amelia and I am six years old. I have only known for one year that I have celiac disease. I miss Oreo biscuits but my mummy makes me some now which I love. I went to a celiac Christmas party and we received Christmas presents and had a lot of gluten-free food. It was nice to be able to eat everything.

There is another girl named Amelia who is also six and has celiac disease too. My mummy also has celiac disease and that makes it easier for me as she has the same food as I do. My brother and sister don't get to have our yummy stuff. My granddad has it as well. He has rice porridge everyday and I had it today with him.

I am going into year one this year. At birthday parties my mummy makes and takes my own cake and lollies to the birthday. My friends mums are kind to me and try to get food I can eat. I have my own jar of lollies at school that the teacher keeps behind her desk. Mummy helps in canteen at school and when she is working she makes me special food so I can feel like the other kids. I usually get gluten-free sausage rolls and pizza bread.

It's not that hard being a celiac and my friends don't mind. 🖊

Amelia's mother, Kate, has written "Welcome To The World Of Celiac Disease," which can be read in Chapter Three, and her grandmother, Janet McMillan, has written "Joining The Celiac Life," which can be read in Chapter Two.

Who Wants a Cookie?

by Kevin Clayton

I live in Phoenix, Arizona and am in the fourth grade. I found out I had celiac disease in December 2002, when I was eight. My mother, father and younger sister all have celiac disease.

At first, everyone has a hard time with celiac disease, and everyone has embarrassing moments with it. My embarrassing moment was when I was at school and a kid asked which I prefer to have at our school party, a cookie or a cupcake. I said I couldn't have either because they have wheat in them. And the other kid said, "There's no wheat in cookies." Everyone who was listening to the conversation said, "Yes, there is wheat in cookies." If I didn't have celiac disease, I could have said I wanted a cupcake and we wouldn't have had this whole discussion. It doesn't embarrass me to have celiac disease, but I am embarrassed by what it can bring about with other kids.

One day at lunch, a kid was waving his cookie around and asking if anybody wanted to eat it. He got his cookie crumbs all over my lunch. I still ate my lunch because it was only a few crumbs and I was really hungry. I knew I shouldn't have eaten the rest of my lunch, but I was really hungry and there wasn't any other food in the cafeteria I could eat. My mom talked to the teacher about it. A few days later she came into my classroom and told the kids how important it was to keep my food gluten-free.

Parties can be difficult too. I have my mom call the people who are doing the school parties and ask what food they are bringing. If it's something like caramel apples, you can talk to them about ingredients. If they are not gluten-free, you can have your mom make up something that is. For birthday parties, I have my mom ask beforehand what foods they are serving. We also ask my teacher to let us know if kids are bringing in treats.

If I can't eat the food, I feel kind of annoyed about it. However, when I come home and there's been food that I couldn't eat, I ask my mom for a treat to make up for what I missed in school.

At first it is a hard diet to stick to, because you're still craving the gluten food. But after half a year, you can't even remember what the other stuff tasted like. It also takes a few weeks for your mom or dad to find some recipes that make food taste good. Then you'll find things you really like to eat.

Kevin's mom, Sue, has written "Living With Celiac Disease: Our First Year," and his younger sister, Angie, has written "My First Gluten-Free Halloween," both of which can be read in Chapter Three.

My Child Has Celiac

Kids Contract The Darndest Things

> Make the best of a sad twist of fate,
> Our children will adapt just great.
> Just watch what they eat,
> Pack a gluten-free treat.
> It insures that their health is first-rate.

What's Wrong With My Daughter?

by Kim Crocker

I am a mother, a teacher, and a student. I home school my nine-year-old daughter on a budget. I read all I can on celiac disease, nutrition and alternative medicine.

Wednesday, November 6, 2002

My eight-year-old daughter had become so ill, she could barely get off the sofa. Between the antacids and the trips to the bathroom, I fought back my tears to read to her from a book. Her symptoms had become so numerous, I did not think anyone would ever figure out what was wrong with her. In the back of my mind I was preparing to lose her.

We were able to get an appointment with a pediatric gastroenterologist. Unfortunately the closest one was a three hour drive and the appointment was still almost a month away. I decided later that afternoon to try the urgent care facility in the town where I live. We had already been there once. When we went during October, for the first time, the doctor had been nice and understanding. She had diagnosed wrong, but at least she had tried something. I planned to take my daughter back there the next day. At the time this was all I could do. I just knew I had to keep trying.

That night, I climbed into bed for another sleepless night and prayed. This time I prayed, not for her to get well, but for God to be with the doctor the next day. I had come to the realization something was very wrong with my daughter. It was not just going to go away. This was not like the ear infections or the viruses of her previous years. This was something different. I prayed for the doctor to be able to decode the symptoms and give this illness a name. Whatever it was, we would deal with it.

Thursday, November 7, 2002

I walked into the doctor's office with my weak, pale, thin daughter. I spewed out all the symptoms one by one for the millionth time. Somehow, this time seemed different. The doctor actually listened to me and was processing each and every symptom as I said it out loud. She walked over to my child and touched her arm. She asked if she had always been thin. I told her yes, but not quite this thin. After twelve doctors and three months, she asked me something that changed our lives forever. "Have you ever heard of celiac disease?"

I had, but didn't know much about it. She did the blood test, which I know now is only a guideline to do further tests. Still worried but hopeful, I went home and attached myself to the computer. I read everything I could about celiac disease. I joined the message board on several Web sites and asked questions. I have learned some of the best information actually comes from celiacs and not doctors.

Friday, November 8, 2002
And so it began. My daughter started on a gluten-free diet. Mind you, becoming gluten-free is not easy and it takes time to get it right. She did better. She experienced less pain, but still couldn't eat.

Saturday, November 9, 2002
Nightmare! She tried to eat a little, but still didn't actually feel hungry. I think she tried to eat to satisfy me. Two bites of food and the whole day went down the drain. You name the stomach medicine and she took it. I was starting to give up. Surely, this can't be it. She was getting very sick all over again.

Sunday, November 10, 2002
She awakened feeling a little better. She tried to eat a little. This time, it hurt a little less than the day before. Still, she wasn't saying she was hungry. Perhaps, this wasn't it. Maybe we were close though.

Monday, November 11, 2002
I was still determined to stick to the diet even if she wasn't that much better. Others on message boards had told me that sometimes it could take as long as a week to see any improvement at all. Also, I had read children tend to suffer the symptoms worse but was warned to be patient because when the diet kicks in, it is somewhat miraculous. I still felt maybe my prayer was about to be answered.

She had been sleepwalking again and awakened on the sofa. I stood in the kitchen sipping my coffee. Suddenly, she popped up and looked around. I thought she was confused by her surroundings by waking up in the wrong place. Once again, I was wrong. However, things were about to start going very right.

She looked at me and said she thought she was hungry. She was as startled as I was. Then she said she was very hungry. I did not know whether to laugh or cry. So, I did both. I pulled out all the important things for a gluten-free breakfast and got busy in the kitchen. I cautiously watched her eat. When she was finished, she needed an antacid. She held it down though. The discomfort went away fairly quick compared to our past episodes. That day, she ate every thirty minutes or so. Also that day, the blood tests came back positive.

One Month Later
When the time came to go to the specialist, we had been gluten-free for almost a month and she had improved quite a bit. The doctor did not seem to believe she could have celiac or that she had truly been gluten-free. After, another doctor came in and subtly questioned us to see if we really knew what we were talking about. He was soon satisfied we did. They wanted to do the biopsy, which meant going down that terrible road we had already been down for three months. She would have to go back to eating gluten for the test. With no biopsy, there would be no official diagnosis. I refused to have my daughter suffer any more and suddenly was in charge of everything. Without a diagnosis, I became the doctor and the dietitian.

The Present
This has not been an easy road, but I think I have risen to the occasion. You never know what you can do until you have

to do it. I recommend strongly getting the proper tests done, but I just could not see my daughter getting that sick again. We just celebrated our first "Gluten-Free Independence Day." In our house it is a holiday. My daughter and I get in the kitchen and play with new recipes. You know, only the sweet ones.

It took us eight months to get her weight back. Slowly one by one, most of the symptoms started to disappear. She still has some minor issues, which I attribute to the length of time she went undiagnosed. The recovery is another story in itself.

She is so active now. Her radio is loud again and she practices cheerleading in my living room. In fact, I am having a hard time writing this because she is chasing stray cats on my front yard in the rain. Next week, she's dragging me off to basketball practice. I can hardly wait. ✍

No Wheat, Rye, Oats, Or Barley

by Amy McKinley

I am the mother of two boys, one six years old and the other six months old. My six-year-old was diagnosed with celiac disease when he was 15 months. There is no celiac disease in either my or my husband's family. Before my son's diagnosis I had never heard of celiac disease.

No wheat, rye, oats, or barley because I am a celiac. That was a song I made up for my 15-month-old sick baby boy. Gluten, never heard of it before 1998. I thought Cheerios, Wheat Thins, and Zweiback were all wholesome foods. But I found out to some babies they are poisons. It all started when Tyler was around seven months of age and first started eating food. He was always long and lean. He also had very fair skin because he was anemic (a symptom of celiac).

At nine plus months he seemed different. Although he remained very thin, he had a distended belly. His coloring was horrible. He was very clingy and we called him "The Blow Out King," due to his explosive bowel movements. We went to the doctors a lot because he had many colds and chronic ear infections. He was losing weight and not growing. The doctors thought his diarrhea was because of all the antibiotics he was taking due to his ear infections. They blamed his crankiness on a possible milk allergy. They weren't overly concerned because after all, he was reaching his big milestones: walking, communicating, etc.

Between 12 and 24 months, he was exhausted all the time and could hardly walk or keep his head up. He never jumped or ran around like other kids his age. He ate very franticly like he never saw food before and kept moving his head. He never stayed still. Yet he was looking so sick and thin. Then he started to vomit after eating, sometimes three to four times a day. On top of that he would have five or more diarrhea diapers.

It was suggested that I take him to a gastrointestinal doctor. We went to Yale New Haven Hospital where they took blood and examined him. The doctor knew right away he was a celiac. We were lucky because the doctor had studied celiac disease while doing his internship.

We needed to do an endoscopy, the only 100% test. Meanwhile we had to keep feeding him gluten because we were told gluten had to be present in the body for a true diagnosis. We were so worried his fragile body wouldn't be able to handle losing anymore fluids. They put him under anesthesia. It was a freaky and scary experience to see my child that way. One hour later the doctor said he had celiac disease.

What a relief finally knowing what was wrong with Tyler and how to handle it. So I started our search for gluten-free food for babies. It was made more complicated because he was also allergic to milk, dairy, soy, and red dye 40. By a lucky coincidence, our pediatrician was treating another child with celiac. So I called the child's mother, crying because I didn't know what to feed Tyler. She invited us to her home where she so graciously put out a gluten-free buffet for him.

It took a lot of trial and error to make sure everything was gluten-free and it has truly paid off. Almost six years later Tyler is in the 95 percentile for height and weight. He has so much energy, sometimes too much, and he is a healthy, happy, smart, and handsome kid. I still call lots of companies to check products since they change ingredients a lot.

It takes time to learn and educate yourself on reading ingredients and understanding where things are derived from. It's very important to make sure all surfaces are free of gluten crumbs. We keep butter, cream cheese, etc for Tyler separate from our own. Tyler has his own pantry and he manages his diet very well at play dates, school, etc. We were just blessed with a second baby boy who we will raise as a celiac too.

All in all, we are very thankful it's a disease that can be controlled by food. ✍

My Little Miracle Girl
by Nick Pierson

My name is Nick Pierson. I believe it is because of my daughter, Nicolette, that I now have a chance to live to a ripe old age (God willing). Her traumatizing celiac diagnosis at such a young age sent me on an inward quest to find out the truth behind my own past and present ailments. This was no easy journey and it was full of pitfalls. But whenever I felt like giving up, I'd think of how bravely my baby girl sat in that hospital bed with those tubes sticking out of her, and my strength would return in abundance.

My little celiac girl
Oh, how I worry about you.
My little 18-month-old,
What is it that ails you,
My little girl?

The bloating,
The crying,
And most horrible of all
The constant throwing up.

If only I could pinpoint it.
It must be my fault.
Why can't I find what ails you,
My little girl?

I was naive to think
You could handle that food.
My little girl,
I'm so sorry.

The grief, oh, the grief.
The doctors diagnose away.
They say not to worry,
You will get better,
My little 20-month-old.

More of the same
And time goes by.
You are still the same,
My little girl.

Your mom cries for you uncontrollably.
Your dad gets angry at them.
How will you feel tomorrow,
My little girl?

What are you thinking?
So small and innocent.
I wish I could take your pain
And make it mine,
My little girl.

I know what I must do,
My little 23-month-old.
I will fight for you
With my heart and soul.
I will make a stand for you,
My little girl.

I will confront my fears
And submit you to more tests.
Oh, how I worry about you,
My little girl.

I'm sorry, so sorry,
That you must go through these tests.
Ignore the tubes and needles if you can,
My little girl.

Please don't cry,
My baby girl.
I promise we will find
What ails you.

Three nights in the hospital,
Waiting, hoping.
Finally they take you
From me and your mom,
My little girl.

I have never been so scared,
So vulnerable,
But the news is great,

You will get better,
My little celiac girl.

You are getting stronger,
My little girl.
You are getting bigger,
My little girl.

Thank you, God, for
My little girl.
I love her so dearly.

Raising A Celiac Child
by Tom Townsend

*I am a 49-year-old resident of Collingswood, New Jersey. I've
been married to my wife, Patti, for 21 years. We have two
daughters, Jessica, who will be 19 and is a freshman in college, and
Kimberly, who is 17 and a senior in high school. I was diagnosed
with celiac disease after many years of classic symptoms. Jessica was
diagnosed shortly thereafter. Ironically my wife, Patti, was
diagnosed in 2002 after suffering for years with multiple symptoms.
So the Townsend household is truly gluten-free, except for the bread
Kim still uses for her lunches.*

*I come from a large family and to date, one sister has been
diagnosed and another sister, who is showing symptoms, is trying the
gluten-free diet to see if her symptoms subside. A niece has also been
diagnosed.*

My wife, Patti, and I may be the exceptions.
We've read a lot of articles about the
difficulties and challenges of raising a child
with celiac disease. For some reason we haven't found it that
difficult. So here's our story.

I was diagnosed with celiac disease in 1996 at age 42. My
diagnosis came the week of Thanksgiving after a difficult
illness and a week in the hospital for emergency surgery on

my intestines (a long story that will not be painfully shared here). After doing some quick Internet research (http://www.celiac.com was then, and still remains today, in our opinion, the best Web site for celiac disease) we found out celiac disease is hereditary and that it would be a good idea to

...we've found it much easier to simply make most family meals completely gluten-free instead of trying to make two sets of meals.

have both of our daughters (ages 10 and 11) tested. Naturally, being the typical 90's parents, we put the blood tests off for several months until we felt guilty enough to have it done in February 1997.

The blood tests confirmed our suspicions about Jessica as they came back positive. We immediately scheduled an endoscopy at Children's Hospital. The results of the biopsy completely confirmed the diagnosis.

Actually, during those few months in which we put off the testing, I was fortunate enough to have done considerable research on the condition via the Internet. I also had time to learn to cook and bake gluten-free. Thus, we avoided the trauma many families feel when a child is diagnosed and the parents are forced to cope with the diagnosis while learning the ins and outs of the diet. We were already halfway toward that objective.

So, what is it really like being parents of a child with celiac disease? Well, we quickly learned several key points that led to a successful adaptation, at least for us. Hopefully they'll prove helpful to you too.

First, we've found it much easier to simply make most

family meals completely gluten-free instead of trying to make two sets of meals. For example, when we have pasta for dinner, it is always gluten-free (Pastariso and Tinkayada are two good ones and can be obtained at Fresh Fields). We recognize that doing it this way is a bit more expensive, but the convenience is well worth it and I dare anyone to taste the difference. The same goes for meatballs or meatloaf, both are made with gluten-free breadcrumbs. Cakes, pies, cookies and muffins are all made with gluten-free flours, even when the cake is for my non-celiac daughter, Kimberly. Patti makes a fantastically delicious and moist chocolate cake that is to die for. (The recipe can be found on the back of Hershey's Cocoa mix container. Just don't forget to add xanthan gum.) In fact, once we

We gave her classroom teacher a bag of candy that could be stored in her drawer in case there were any surprise treats she did not know about in advance.

were diagnosed, all wheat flours were banned from the house, as we never wanted to put ourselves in the position of accidentally using the wrong flours!

Of course, not everything in the house is gluten-free as the cost would be prohibitive, not to mention unfair to Patti and Kim. For example, there are non gluten-free cereals, breads (for lunches), store bought cookies and pretzels, as well as beer (the one and only item I still miss!).

What about Jessie? What has it been like for her? Well, we quickly learned that as parents we had to adapt, be more flexible and most importantly, plan ahead. When diagnosed, Jessie was in sixth grade so she was still of the age when kids are known to bring in cakes, cookies, and other goodies to celebrate birthdays. Or maybe a teacher would celebrate a class' good performance by having a pizza party. So what do you do?

Well, we first sat with each of Jessie's teachers and explained the situation. We gave her classroom teacher a bag of candy that could be stored in her drawer in case there were any surprise treats she did not know about in advance. Was it the same for Jes? Frankly, no, but at least while the other kids were eating donut holes Jes could have a bag of M&M's. For those occasions when we knew in advance (with help from the teacher) about a scheduled treat, we would always try to duplicate that treat. On the many days this occurred I would bet many in the class did not suspect anything out of the ordinary. This is perfect for the celiac child.

We learned early on how to make a great gluten-free pizza. Recipes can be found in Bette Hagman's and other gluten-free cookbooks, or mixes can be purchased from the Gluten-Free Pantry and other mail order vendors. We've made pizzas in advance and wrapped them in aluminum foil. Jes really doesn't mind eating cold pizza, as again, her main objective is to have pizza with everyone else and not to appear to be different. We've made many, many pizzas for birthday parties, class trips, class parties, sleepovers, etc., and Jes is able to fit in, making it all worthwhile from our perspective.

Speaking of class trips, you really have to think ahead and plan to provide the proper gluten-free environment for your child. Trips that last a full day or even overnight require the most work as numerous meals are involved. We have always coordinated with the teacher/leader of the trip to find out exactly where they planned to eat. If it was McDonald's, well that was easy as we only had to provide Jes with a gluten-free hamburger roll (yes, we even make those) and she knows to order a quarter pounder without the roll. Otherwise, we spend time on the phone calling the restaurant and speaking with the chef or manager as to what meals were being served. Most times they are very willing to help you out and prepare something separate for your child. We try to keep it real simple and ask for a piece of plain grilled chicken (no flour dredging please!). While many may frown and say that doesn't sound very appealing, take note that Jes is thrilled and I would suspect your child would be too.

> *If I could give any final advice to parents of celiac children it would be to know the diet completely, learn to bake if you don't already know how, plan, and be willing to adapt...*

Breakfast is generally pretty easy, as scrambled eggs are always fine for Jes. For one excursion we actually took complete meals to her field trip, as we were not comfortable with what we were hearing from the chef. The one thing we have found to be amazing is that as time goes by, Jes has learned more and more about the diet and has developed a confidence level which allows her to not lean on us for every food related decision. The last few trips, Jes has actually shown little concern about her food and has said to us, "I'm not worried about the food, I'll find something to eat." And she does, since many places have self help salad bars. Jes realizes at worst she'll have to improvise and eat a salad or a yogurt but that it's only one meal and she's not as concerned about feeling left out or different.

All of Jessie's friends know about her condition, as do her friends' parents. Most are accommodating and have gluten-free snacks on hand for Jes to eat. Jessica's best friend has even declined snacks for herself when she realizes there were no gluten-free snacks for Jes to eat. Now that's a friend!

Some thoughts from Jessica's perspective:

* Initially, she felt there was nothing for her to eat, but she slowly found there were lists available of the many gluten-free foods and candies she could eat.

* Sometimes she has to go without snacks at school and this can be hard when surprised by non gluten-free snacks.

* She realizes the burden of finding out about snacks at school is now on her shoulders and if she fails to tell us about it ahead of time, she has to do without.

* She has learned to cook and bake some gluten-free foods. She made a great German Apple Cake and took it to her German class in school. The class devoured it.

*   Most importantly of all, Jes knows that celiac disease is only a part of her. Jessica doesn't consider herself a celiac, simply a 14-year old-girl who just happens to have some diet restrictions.

With Jes now entering high school, we realize we have most of the formula down pat. Home-made gluten-free bread for lunches, gluten-free snacks and a daughter who is learning to function gluten-free on her own. Next step...college! Yikes.

Parting Words:

I truly feel blessed to have been diagnosed with celiac disease. First and foremost the diagnosis allowed me to feel completely healthy for probably the first time in my life. Secondly, it allowed me, as a parent, to lead the way for my daughter as she was going through the gluten-free adjustment. In many ways our path has been easier with Jes because of my diagnosis.

If I could give any final advice to parents of celiac children it would be to know the diet completely, learn to bake if you don't already know how, plan, and be willing to adapt, but most of all, smile and enjoy the years you have with your children as they quickly grow to high school and college aged kids!

Postscript:

The above was written four years ago. Jessica entered Gettysburg College as a freshman this September and she continues to thrive. Much has happened in the past four years as is the case with all teenagers experiencing high school: plays, field hockey, dances, jobs, and more. Jes has learned a truly valuable lesson and that is a simple condition like celiac disease is no more than a speed bump in life, easily navigated with the right attitude and outlook. More companies are also producing gluten-free foods.

We are extremely blessed to have found such a great school in Gettysburg College. They are very accommodating in the cafeteria and Jes has her own supply of breads, rolls, pizza shells, cookies, and brownies waiting for her in the freezer in the kitchen. The chefs all know Jes and go out of their way to make sure she is not left out and has plenty to eat.

As she has done since the beginning and as all of us with this condition know, you must learn to ask questions when it comes to knowing how your food is prepared. Jes is happy, and we, as parents, are not only happy but also relieved to know our daughter not only knows how to take care of herself, but that others can and do extend themselves to make sure she is not excluded. ✍

She's Going To Do Just Fine
by *Patricia Vlamis*

I am the mother of Mary, a five-year-old with celiac disease for whom I enjoy making special gluten-free foods. I produce a newsletter for the Greater New Haven Children's Celiac Group in Connecticut, as well as being the co-chairperson of the group. I am a photographer with my own business, PMV Images.com, in which I create custom cards and invitations using photographs. My husband John and I have another daughter, Christina, three, who does not have celiac but enjoys gluten-free cookies as much as her sister.

In October of 2001, my oldest daughter, Mary, was diagnosed with celiac disease. She was just three years old at the time, old enough to remember eating foods that tasted good but made her tummy hurt, yet young enough to not have too many established routines that revolved around food related activities such as pizza parties.

As her mom, I began the quest every mother of a celiac goes through when their child is first diagnosed. I scoured the Internet and cookbooks for recipes and spent a small fortune at the health food stores buying alternative flours and anything I could find labeled gluten-free.

Slowly, I established a routine and found what Mary's likes and dislikes were. We discovered what tasted good and what tasted like sawdust. After a month on the gluten-free diet Mary began to gain weight and was growing! It was working. Somewhere along the way I accepted this would be her lifestyle and we would have to deal with whatever obstacles we faced in following a gluten-free diet together.

The summer she was four she attended a week long day camp. I contacted the camp director to find out what the snack would be for each day. Conscious of not wanting her to feel different from the other kids, I tried my best to provide her with gluten-free equivalents of what they were having. One day they were making jelly sandwiches and then cutting shapes in them with cookie cutters. I told Mary I would send her bread and jelly to camp with her so she could make sandwiches also. She looked me straight in the eye and said, "I can't use the cutters the other kids use, they will have their wheat all over it." I couldn't believe she picked that out so quickly, even before I had thought of it. I knew then I wouldn't have to worry about her too much when she was away from me. It is so important to teach our kids not to be shy about asking if a certain food is something they can have. The fact that she knows enough to ask gives me a certain level of comfort.

Although she is still small, I try to include her when I make special gluten-free items, such as pizza or cookies. I try to stress to her that she will have to be responsible for her food someday and she needs to learn how to prepare it.

A Gluten-Free "Baker's Dozen" And Then Some...

by Melonie Katz

Melonie has also written the introduction to this book "What Is Celiac," and the piece "I Can't Believe They Said That," which can be read in Chapter 12.

It's a misconception that celiac disease is rare and that doctors will see only a few celiac cases during their careers. Luckily, increased research has contributed to the expanded awareness of celiac disease for medical professionals and for the general population. To reach our toddler's final diagnosis of celiac disease, it took one persistent set of parents and twenty-four medical personnel, including a multitude of pediatricians, radiologists, emergency room physicians, a dietician, two pediatric gastroenterologists, and a very long four months.

Here's our story: Our 15-month-old talking toddler began experiencing intractable diarrhea and periodic episodes of vomiting that kept reappearing. I was told it was probably a "viral thing" and she would get better. I was basically dismissed. However, on the eighth straight day of her symptoms continuing to worsen, we made yet another visit to the pediatrician. We went home again without answers to the cause of her ongoing illness. That evening, I surfed the Internet and discovered research on celiac disease and some information on Danna Korn, the founder of R.O.C.K. (Raising Our Celiac Kids). After learning just a little bit about celiac disease that evening, I was convinced our toddler had it due to her long list of celiac related symptoms: diarrhea, vomiting, weight loss, loss of muscle mass,

> *The doctors were baffled and many of them would come by to visit her just to look, and I could hear them down the hallway talking in amazement that they did not know what could possibly be wrong.*

irritability, excessive crying and screaming, distended abdomen, and her eventually intolerance of milk products. I started my mission that evening: to find the "cause" of our daughter's illness and to get proper testing and an accurate diagnosis. It took four long months of numerous visits to various doctors who all believed that celiac was not likely and never tested for it.

In the meantime, I kept a food diary on our daughter's diet, maintained an "I & O" sheet (intake/outtake) for months and even delivered stool samples to the doctor routinely. On a daily basis, we eventually reached about twenty explosive diarrhea diapers and several episodes of projectile vomiting. The vomiting usually happened during sleeping hours, when her abdomen was "relaxed." She went from a size four diaper to a size one diaper, and the size one eventually would not stay on due to the lack of muscle mass to hold it on. I used a bread bag tie or a plastic produce bag clip to help keep her diaper from falling off. During these four long months of many visits to the doctor, she stopped talking, had no interest in playing or eating and slept a lot.

After four visits to the first pediatrician, she was eventually put on a "Pedialyte only liquid diet," and we were told to continue with a bland diet such as the BRAT (bananas, rice, apples, and toast) diet and plain things like crackers or noodles. Her condition worsened, as you can imagine. Giving her the toxic gluten containing foods continued to make her worse. She continued to lose weight. She went from 26 pounds to 16 pounds. Her hips would nearly pop out of the socket during the frequent diaper changes due to her lack of muscle mass. Her body was not absorbing any nutrients at all and she was becoming malnourished. Dark circles began to appear under her eyes and her face looked sunken in.

Eventually, a visit to the emergency room and an admitting diagnosis of "Failure to Thrive" began to get us in the right direction. The doctors were baffled and many of them would come by to visit her just to look, and I could hear them down the hallway talking in amazement that they did not know what could possibly be wrong. We were asked if we had visited any third world countries or if we had been exposed to any untreated water (since we had just made a move from the East Coast to the West Coast). We were asked to sign a release to test for HIV and more. The doctors began talk of contacting the CDC (Centers for Disease Control in Atlanta) for more direction. They tested her for hepatitis, and even suspected she may have had a bad reaction to hepatitis vaccine (that was given several months prior). She was tested for rotavirus, giardia (traveler's diarrhea), stomach tumors, and a multitude of other conditions. An ultrasound was done to see if there were any masses or cysts. They even did a fat/stool test and a salt test for cystic fibrosis before they would test for celiac. Finally, on her third day in the hospital, the Chief of Pediatrics seemed to believe that maybe this zany mom may be on to something. They did a celiac blood panel and the results were very high. We were finally on the path to a real diagnosis. She remained in the hospital for a few more days for monitoring and to continue IV fluids due to dehydration. We had to keep her on a diet containing gluten, so the endoscopy results would be accurate. Her "sickness" continued until the day of the endoscopy, which was done at the local Children's Hospital.

Immediately after the endoscopy, I started her on a gluten-free diet as we waited for those results. Within 48 hours of the gluten-free diet, her diarrhea and vomiting were completely gone. She was like a new child, with a new reason to live, to play, have fun, and interact. The next week, the biopsy results confirmed celiac disease and we have gone forward with a positive outlook ever since. After months of intestinal healing, she is now able to tolerate dairy products. During her extreme illness, her intestines had developed some ulcerous areas due to the toxicity of the gluten and required months of medication, as well as a vitamin D and calcium supplement. Miraculously, the gluten-free diet catapulted her into great health.

Our loving toddler has adjusted well to the gluten-free diet and we have ventured into the gluten-free lifestyle with welcome arms. The bright side of things is, she required no surgeries and no lifelong medications. We said goodbye to most convenience foods and most toddler friendly foods, and embraced the new diet change to healthy gluten-free foods. She has been gluten-free for over a year and has almost finished her speech therapy sessions to make up for the time that her body was focused on trying to survive. Her tenacity has inspired each of our family members and we know that nothing will hold her back.

We are fortunate that our experience was only four months because in our country, most people unknowingly live with celiac disease for an average of ten or eleven years before getting a proper diagnosis. Through our persistent efforts and the tenacity of a few doctors, we found the reason for our daughter's sickness and are grateful to everyone who helped in our journey to good health. Thankfully, many in the celiac community have helped pave the way for others, and we hope we can continue to pave that path too.

One Less Thing
To Worry About

by Sharla Wiatt

Sharla has also written "Be Positive," which can be read in Chapter Four.

A van came through our neighborhood and two men in the back of the van asked the neighborhood kids to come with them. They told them they had ice cream and yummy treats for them in the van. I was worried how my four-year-old daughter would have responded if they had asked her. I told her the story and asked her what she would have done. She replied, "Oh mom, of course I wouldn't have gone. The treats probably had gluten or dairy in them!"

I'll Make A Deal With You, God

by Marilyn Carr

I live in Gig Harbor, Washington. I am retired from a career working for various county prosecutors where I specialized in assisting victims of serious crimes.

I am very proud of my 22-year-old daughter, Ashley. I say proud because she has celiac disease and has accepted her "condition" and "limitations." It has made her a strong advocate for herself and others whose lives do not fit into a perfect box.

As a mother of a celiac daughter, I have often spoken these words to God. I have asked God to give me her pain and discomfort and just let her live her life like a normal, healthy, pain free 22-year-old has the right to. My prayers have not yet been answered.

My pregnancy with Ashley was marked with morning sickness for five months, sinusitis, and back pain for three months. According to my doctor's calculations, she was exactly two hours and three minutes over due. She was full term, yet, they referred to her as a "preemie" as she weighed five pounds, seven ounces. I remember feeling angry and resentful every time the nursing staff referred to her as a preemie. It was as if I did something wrong and she was not healthy. In the first few hours of her life they decided she was breaking down her enzymes too quickly, something that should not have happened for several more months. It was my obstetrician who assured me this was common in low birth weight babies and it was nothing to worry about. In addition, I had the RH negative factor but had not experienced any problems.

Early on, Ashley did not tolerate any formula that was not soy based. She was prone to ear infections and the doctor kept her on a maintenance dose of Bactrim, an antibacterial combination drug. I noticed each time she was fed cow milk based formula, she almost always got an ear infection. Her pediatrician did not seem impressed, but my own allergist thought I was pretty sharp for catching it.

We moved to Iowa when Ashley was just starting the second grade. That year, she had strep throat nine times. Finally, her doctor sent the throat swab to disease control and it was determined she had a strain of strep that was quite rare in Iowa. She subsequently had the same infection at least once a year for the next five years. The summer before her fourth grade she was ill with pneumonia. In the fourth grade she was seen by her first specialist, a pediatric gastroenterologist for her stomach problems. She would have bouts of diarrhea and stomach pain, often before special events. After a series of tests, our minds were put to rest. We simply had a daughter who "strives to be perfect and this is how she deals with stress." What a relief. Of course now I realize, that was probably the beginning of her problems and I did not have the knowledge to even consider a second opinion. After all, she had just been seen by a pediatric gastroenterologist that was brought in from Omaha.

As she grew older, her symptoms worsened. At 14, we took her to an adult gastroenterologist who diagnosed her as having irritable bowel syndrome. I was unsure of this diagnosis and sought a second opinion at our nationally recognized children's hospital. After several biopsies and lab reports, she was diagnosed

> *Had we had this diagnosis while she was younger, I believe her life would have been very different. We didn't and she suffered greatly.*

with eosinophilic gastroenteritis. She was put on several medications and she was fed through a pic line. Again, we accepted the diagnosis and followed the treatment.

Ashley's high school years are almost a blur to me. She suffered greatly with continual pain, vomiting, and diarrhea. On a daily basis, she was ill, often sleeping on the bathroom floor during the night. Her attendance suffered and so did her school work. It did not take long for her "friends" to stop calling. Ashley would not be invited to social events. I mean can you blame them? Who wants to go out to dinner with a friend who gets sick and has to go home? I was very depressed and would usually start crying as my front wheels drove over the curb in the morning heading to work. I cried because all I wanted was for my daughter to feel like a healthy, normal teenager, go to school and just live her life.

It looked like trying to get help from the school was going to be a hurdle. Then, through a friend, I was told about 504 plans and the 1972 Disabilities Act. The discovery of the 504 plan and the Disabilities Act is what it took for me to put on my "advocate cape" to do battle with the school. I wish I could tell you the staff was considerate, understanding, and helpful, but I can't. Frankly, the counselor did not want to do any extra work and actually said so during a meeting. At one point my husband almost had to be physically restrained from coming to blows with this counselor. I had to advise the staff my daughter was different than others at her school. Ashley would be going to college and we needed their help. She was not going to drop out of high school and work at the local fast food restaurant for the rest of her life.

On the surface they were delightful and offered to do whatever it took. Without spending a great deal of time on those headaches, let me just use the phrase, "out of sight out of mind..." That would pretty much cover the next two years.

It got so bad Ashley finally dropped out of high school. She sat for the GED and did very well. Then she attended classes at the local community college. Many semesters she could only take two classes in order to plan her schedule around her diarrhea and illness. But she stuck with it and it paid off. We are so proud of her and were thrilled to attend her college graduation this past May.

It was not until June of 2002 that the Mayo Clinic diagnosed her with celiac sprue. I had taken her there along with her fiancé, Bryan. Receiving that diagnosis was wonderful. Yes, wonderful. At last we had a correct diagnosis and something that could hopefully be put into remission. No surgeries, drugs, or pills, just a proper diet.

Had we had this diagnosis while she was younger, I believe her life would have been very different. We didn't and she suffered greatly. However, today she is a strong woman who takes control of her health issues and has the confidence to deal head on with anyone in the medical field she does not think is providing adequate care for her.

It is very difficult to deal with your chronically sick child. If your child or loved one has this disease you must have a heart big enough to become a celiac with them. Don't eat the 'wrong' foods in their presence. Find out what foods are gluten-free and eat them, cook with gluten-free ingredients, or at least, have food available they can eat. Think about it. How easily could you give up fast foods, pastries, candies and such? Starting now, give it all up for a week. Attempt to walk in their shoes for a short period of time. Oh, and by the way, add bloating, cramping, and diarrhea to your daily routine, and don't forget the need for a bathroom within a few feet.

It is a small thing to ask of friends, family, and restaurants to have food items available to all persons who have special food needs. This disease is thought to be grossly under diagnosed. My guess is that more people have been misdiagnosed with other conditions than correctly diagnosed with celiac sprue. The good news is that if the strict diet is kept to, it should never be life threatening, simply life altering.

As a parent I can tell you the hardest part of having a sick child is to let them come to terms with their illness. That is, to take responsibility for what they eat and don't eat. They have to find it within themselves to live with the disease and figure out what they have to do to make life tolerable. 🖎

Marilyn's daughter, Ashley Reynolds-Rasmussen, has written "One Molecule," which can be read in Chapter Four.

Making It Easier For Our Children

No Kidding

> *There is nothing that I wouldn't do,*
> *To take care of my child with sprue.*
> *I'll relearn how to cook,*
> *Just give me a book.*
> *If it helps I'll eat gluten-free too.*

Anything For Our Children
by Kathleen Johe

I would like to give thanks to my husband and son, for without them, I'd be lost. Also to my friends at the Marx Bros. Cafe, UAA Culinary Arts, Chinatown YMCA, and Allen & Peterson, from whom I have learned so much about food and life. Thanks, of course, to my family. When I need to laugh, cry, scream, or just be, no one else will do. Lastly, thank you so very much to those who have provided so much information regarding the disease and how to live with it, without your contributions, we would all be lost.

First of all, I should tell all of you I am not a diagnosed celiac. My beautiful, wonderful, inspiring now three-year-old son is. Yes, after his diagnosis, we, like many celiacs wondered where he got it from, since it is hereditary. My mother and I have suffered with digestive problems most of our lives, so it seemed easy to assume it came from me. I was tested, via blood test only, and the results were negative. But no matter, that is not what this story is about. This is not a story about struggles with getting a proper diagnosis, or dealing with dieticians and doctors who know less than you do about the disease. This story is about my journey as the mother of a celiac.

I should tell those of you who are struggling with diagnosis, to keep your chins up. Doctors are becoming more and more aware of the disease every day. My son, Bryce, was one of the lucky ones. He was sick, my God, was he sick. But compared to most, his diagnosis was relatively quick and his recovery was even quicker. He was diagnosed at a tender age one.

We had been on a family vacation to California when he became very ill on the flight home. After we landed, we headed directly to the emergency room. Bryce could barely breathe. The initial diagnosis of his immediate symptoms was croup coupled with a respiratory infection called RSV (respiratory syncytial virus). The combination was caused by a virus and can often be deadly. The onset was so quick, only a matter of hours. But the track of the infection was curbed and my son was on the road to recovery within a matter of days. Or so we thought.

While the symptoms of his infection disappeared with the antibiotics, others began presenting themselves. Not only digestive issues, but behavioral issues as well. Bryce was always moody, and because of the severe acidity of his bowel movements, he would develop burns on his tender skin within minutes. We were in the doctor's office quite often in those next weeks and months, and we received the same diagnosis I'm sure you all received, irritable bowel syndrome. But, no, my son did not have irritable bowel syndrome. After a few months of making at least 10 to 15 diarrhea diaper changes a day and slathering on every rash cream known to mankind, the doctor finally took a blood test. Yup, it was celiac disease, brought out of dormancy by the severe viral infection.

When I went home, I went on-line immediately and searched for celiac information. At least I can say there is a wealth of information out there. You need only to look for it. I learned all I could and then went to the grocery store armed with the safe and forbidden foods list from celiac.com. That first trip to the store was not one I am likely to ever forget. It seemed like there was nothing, I mean nothing, other than Fritos, vegetables and meat. While

My first gluten-free cake was fabulous when I pulled it out of the oven. Ten minutes later it could have been used for skeet shooting.

I realize now that veggies and meat alone are versatile to say the least, at the time I kept thinking, how is my son ever going to get used to this? What will happen when he is invited to his first birthday party, sleepover, or goes on his first date. What will he eat? Will he eat a chicken breast and a broccoli floret? I don't think so. I made a vow, right then and there. My son would have it all. There would be no, "Sorry, he's allergic," or "No thanks, it could kill me." Instead, he would be the one asking, "Would you like to try some of mine?"

At that time I was in a computer engineering program in college. I was in my second semester, but I knew what I had to do. I switched my major, and went into the culinary program. To be honest, for me, it wasn't really that much of a hardship. Cooking had always been a passion of mine, and I'm sure all you readers will understand what I mean when I say that food is power. It can make you smile, sigh, giggle, leave you wanting more and the lack of it can make you cry. People fall in love, break up, meet others, get engaged, and make or break business deals over fantastic meals. Sometimes mealtime is the only time families get together. So you see, for me, education in the art and science of food was the only way.

I learned the proper techniques to make every dish from sweet to savory. I learned the science of baking and why gluten is such an important ingredient in many goods. In turn, I learned when it is necessary, how it can be substituted and when it

My son has been gluten-free for nearly two years now and is off the charts in size for his age bracket.

can be omitted all together. I learned all this because I wanted to make a muffin for my son, that didn't double as hockey puck. I wanted to taste gluten-free bread that didn't sandblast the enamel off my molars. So I endured two years of tyrannical and moody chefs, because they were brilliant. I waited tables in restaurants for free because it fulfilled degree requirements and I took a job for nine dollars an hour at a sweaty little kitchen in an upscale café.

During my free time, what little there was of it, I experimented. My first gluten-free cake was fabulous when I pulled it out of the oven. Ten minutes later it could have been used for skeet shooting. So I wasn't savvy in the ways of gluten-free cooking just yet. But I was getting better.

My second try was much better. I had read an excerpt from one of Bette Hagman's gluten-free cookbooks and learned with gluten-free baked goods I should lower the temperature and increase the bake time. This sets the structure so it won't fall like a rock off a cliff after it comes out of the oven.

I experimented with different flours and learned to feel them between my fingers before deciding what best use they would have. All this time I was feeding my son and husband with my attempts. Cookies were easily mastered, cakes a close second. Breads are still a work in progress; I think my standards are very high. Bagels and donuts are on the back burner for the time being and pizza crust is the current project. I like some of the published recipes, but for the most part, I seem to have better luck inventing my own.

Now that I have my degree, I have quite a collection of recipes and have begun teaching gluten-free cooking classes. This first class I taught went more than an hour longer than scheduled. No one wanted to leave. Our city has no support groups, so for some of the people it was the first time they had ever been in the same room with another celiac. One lovely lady had not had cake, cookies, or bread of any kind in more than six years! She made me want to cry. We made a decadent chocolate cake, buttermilk rolls, snicker doodle cookies, and chicken parmesan. It was incredible. We talked about different flours, cooking techniques, and mainstream products that are gluten-free. I learned so much more from these people who have been living the life for years than I did with a thousand Internet searches. And I was supposed to be the teacher!

That brings us to the present. My son has been gluten-free for nearly two years now and is off the charts in size for his age bracket. He is a healthy and handsome little man, who will be breaking the ladies hearts sooner than I would like. He is still learning about his diet, and why he can't have certain foods unless Mommy makes them, but he takes it all in stride. He is resilient, as only a child can be.

This is the point where I would like to offer a little advice for those struggling parents of celiac babies. Don't be afraid to experiment. That's how we learn, by making mistakes. Spend as much one-on-one time with your kitchen as possible. The more you do now, the less you will need to do later. Keep notes on what you have learned so you don't make the same mistake twice. Don't limit yourself to what you can buy but also don't feel like you must make everything from scratch either. There are some really good gluten-free products out there. Eating out is not impossible, but be strong. Don't take any attitude from servers or chefs who don't understand, or think you are just on a low carbohydrate diet. I recommend making up a note card with a list of all things you or your child cannot have and keeping it with you. Give it to the server and have them take it to the chef so they can make a recommendation.

In conclusion, I would just like to say, don't be a slave to your diet, or that of your child's. Yes, food is power, but it is a power you can control. Take everyday one step at a time and love life for the gifts it brings, not the things it takes away. Have faith and someday there may be a cure, but in the meantime, concentrate on yourself and your child, and who knows, maybe when a cure is found, we won't really need it anymore. ✍

Baby Turkey

by Susan Hodges

> *Our family joined the celiac ranks about five years ago when our youngest child, Hannah Rose, was diagnosed with celiac disease. Her symptoms began shortly after her second birthday, with a diagnosis two years later. At four years of age she weighed 19 pounds. The same weight as when she was only one-year-old. She looked like "death warmed over."*
>
> *Today, five years later, she is one of my heroes. She regularly stares down cookies, birthday cakes, and all manner of "surprise" gluten opportunities. I recently underwent abdominal surgery which will result in many gastric limitations. I can only hope I will be as true to myself as my daughter has been these last five years.*
>
> *Blessings, Susan Hodges, Stockton, California. Mom to Hannah Rose, now age nine.*

Since holiday time poses many unique problems for celiacs, I thought I would share the way we did Thanksgiving last year for a large out-of-town family gathering. My main concern was our then eight-year-old daughter, who is the only celiac in the family.

My mom purchased a regular turkey for the larger feast and a Cornish game hen for our daughter. The game hen is now forever known as the "baby turkey" in our family. Mom also bought brown rice and wild rice from Trader Joe's. I brought some gluten-free mild Italian sausage, onion, celery, garlic, and parsley. I made up a stuffing recipe from these ingredients. The salad, vegetables, and Jello salad were all gluten-free (except the rolls, of course). Lastly, we made pumpkin custard from the excess pumpkin pie filling.

Well our daughter was the hit of the children's table. She beamed with pride as cousins, brothers, sisters, and grandparents admired her "baby turkey". She ate well that evening and enjoyed herself. Her grandfather (my dad) couldn't stop raving about the stuffing I made up, so I left the recipe as best I could remember it and he made more the next day before we left.

This year all the children wanted their own "baby turkey" and the birds (large and small) will all use the rice/Italian sausage stuffing instead of the regular one we always made.

You can find Susan's recipe for "Italian Sausage Stuffing" in Chapter 11.

Take The Fight
To The Enemy

by Lieutenant Colonel Michael Heidt

My name is Michael "Max" Heidt, and I am in the US Air Force, stationed at European Command (EUCOM) Headquarters, in Stuttgart, Germany. My daughter, Jessica, has been a type 1 diabetic since age six. She is an amazing young girl and her sister (Brittany), mom, and I support her 100%. We feed off her optimism and positive attitude towards life, despite its challenges.

My daughter, Jessica, has been a type 1 diabetic since age six, so lifestyle changes and discipline are no strangers to this amazing girl (now 12). Blood work in August 2003 indicated an elevation in antigens which classified her as a "borderline" risk for celiac. A biopsy was completed in September 2003 with no signs of the disease. Since Jessica has a quarterly endocrinologist appointment as part of her diabetes care, we anticipate re-testing in spring/summer 2004 with a second biopsy as necessary. Considering the fact that elevated antigens levels are usually indicative of celiac, we have used the past few months to educate ourselves and have even ordered some gluten-free goods on-line in order to taste test. The family has slowly but surely introduced itself to the challenges associated with a gluten-free diet (in the event it becomes a reality in the future).

At first, the news of celiac was a bit intimidating and overwhelming. I felt sorry for Jessica and was angry that she had yet another cross to bear. I personally dwelt on the hardships that would follow (what to eat, what not to eat, how we would travel, etc.). I wanted to take the problem from Jessica, but realized that was unrealistic and that my thoughts were becoming fatalistic and irrational. Slowly but surely and with the grace of God, I grew more comfortable with the issue, realizing the situation could be more dire. So instead, I started to focus daily on the myriad of blessings I (we) have despite life's unfortunate challenges.

Instead of wallowing in self pity, it is far healthier (and more critical) to accept the situation (which cannot be reversed) and redirect attention and energy into ways of making life work! The tools are there and once I accepted the fact and changed my mental/spiritual focus, the pain disappeared and my solutions reappeared.

Take the fight to the enemy!

Gluten-Free Play Materials

by Lindsay Amadeo

I am the parent of two celiac kids, Joe, age nine, and Sam, age six. My husband, Gerard, is also celiac. We are grateful to those who have walked this path before us and shared their tips and experiences to make our experience just a bit easier.

Stringing cereal and pasta, and playing with play dough are big parts of toddler/preschoolers days. And of course kids that age put their hands in their mouths constantly, so the items they play with have to be gluten-free. So I searched and experimented a bit and came up with the following that I'd like to share. Just a note, you can add Kool Aid to the play dough for color, and it also smells great.

Here is a list of gluten-free play materials along with recipes for play dough and paper mache:
* Beeswax.
* Elmer's products - All are gluten-free, except for washable paste.
* Ross' white glue stick, glue stick, and school glue.
* Polymer clay

Play Dough #1

Ingredients:

    1 pound box baking soda
    1 cup cornstarch
    1¼ cups cold water

Directions:

    *Mix the baking soda and corn starch.
    *Add the water and cook over medium heat 10-15 minutes (until mixture resembles mashed potatoes).
    *Put on a plate and cover with a damp cloth.

Play Dough #2

Ingredients:

    ½ cup white rice flour
    ½ cup cornstarch
    ½ cup salt
    2 teaspoons cream of tartar
    1 cup water
    1 teaspoon oil
    food coloring

Directions:

    *Mix all ingredients together in a pan.
    *Cook on low heat for 3 minutes until it forms a ball.

Play Dough #3

Ingredients:
  1 cup salt
  ½ cup cornstarch
  ½ cup boiling water

Directions:
  *Mix all three ingredients in a pan and cook over a low heat, stirring constantly.
  *Knead smooth when cool.

Paper Mache #1

Ingredients:
  ½ cup gluten-free flour
  ¼ teaspoon xanthan gum
  2 cups cold water
  2 cups boiling water
  3 tablespoons sugar

Directions:
  *Mix the flour, xanthan gum, and cold water.
  *Add the mixture to boiling water and return to a boil.
  *Remove from heat and add the sugar.
  *Let it cool and thicken.

Paper Mache #2

Ingredients:
> 1 cup gluten-free flour
> 1 teaspoon xanthan gum
> water

Directions:
> *Mix the gluten-free flour and the xanthan gum.
> *Keep adding up to 3 cups of water until all the lumps are gone.
> *Bring mixture to a boil and then let cool.
> *Dip strips of paper into paste mixture scraping the excess with your fingers.
> *Layer the paste covered strips on the project.

Edible Clay #1

Ingredients:
> 2 cups peanut butter
> 1 cup honey
> 2½ cups powdered milk
> 1 cup powdered sugar

Directions:
> *Mix all the ingredients with a strong mixer.

Edible Clay #2

Ingredients:

1/3 cup margarine
1/2 teaspoon salt
1/3 cup corn syrup
1 teaspoon gluten-free vanilla
1 pound powdered sugar

Directions:

*Knead all the ingredients and add food coloring if desired.
*Keep the mixture in the refrigerator.

Sample Letter To School Teachers

by Lindsay Amadeo

Lindsay has also submitted "Gluten-Free Play Materials," which appears earlier in this chapter.

The following is a letter I developed and sent to my child's preschool teachers prior to the start of the year. Please feel free to adapt it for your needs.

Date

Dear (Teacher),

We are delighted to spend a full year with you and look forward to having Joe and Sam in your class. We can't wait to watch them blossom in your room.

As you may remember from last year, Joe and Sam have celiac disease and must follow a medically restricted diet. Over the past several years we have found the most important thing to help them manage their condition, without feeling excluded, is good communication between the teacher, the kids, Gerard, and myself so we can prepare alternatives for them. If we can talk ahead of time about food related projects, birthdays, holidays, and field trips, I can either suggest a particular brand or substitution that may work for all the kids, or I will send something for Joe and Sam to enjoy while the rest of the class eats what they have prepared. Please don't hesitate to call me at any time to let me know what you are planning, to check to see if something is okay for them, and to let me know how I can help.

In past years, we brought a snack tub for everyday and special occasion treats that worked well. Joe and Sam made their selections from the tub and we replenished often. If that works for you, I will bring one again this year. I am happy to do whatever I can to make things easiest for you and to help Joe and Sam feel included.

Another thing that worked well last year was getting a list of parent sign-ups for holiday parties and a class birthday list. On those days I gave the kids the choice of bringing a special treat or eating from their box. They both seemed to do well having more control over how they wanted to manage the social situation. If it is possible, I'd like to do this again as it helps Joe and Sam take some responsibility for managing their own diet.

Attached is a list of products, by brand name, they can have. All fresh fruits and vegetables, peanuts in the shell, and white milk are safe. The safety of processed foods and juices is complicated and depends entirely on the brand. Safe food can become "contaminated" if it comes into contact with something like crumbs on a table or a knife that was used to spread something on crackers. They will need to lay down a napkin or something at the snack counter.

The kids have different reactions if they eat something unsafe. Joe has no symptoms, although eating gluten prevents him from growing normally. If Sam is exposed to gluten, he will vomit or have stomach pain within 12-24 hours and very loose stools. He will need to use the bathroom urgently if he has eaten something he shouldn't have. Gerard and I will certainly pick him up from school if you notice him holding his stomach or mentioning that it hurts. The pain only lasts for the day, however, the stools will continue to be loose for up to a week. We appreciate knowing of any time they may have been exposed to gluten so we can watch for symptoms and use it as a learning opportunity. Both kids are knowledgeable about safe and unsafe foods, but can be misled when a trusted adult tells them they can have something. For example, they might ask if something is okay, and the adult, thinking they are asking for permission to eat it, doesn't realize they are asking about the safety of the item and says "okay."

Celiac is similar to an allergy in that they must avoid all foods and contact with materials that contain wheat, rye, barley, oats, and their derivatives. Without contact with these products, both kids are fine and can participate in all activities. However, even a trace of gluten will cause serious damage. They can also react from skin contact with gluten. Play dough, paper mache, stringing cereal or pasta, some glues and paints, licking stickers or envelopes, etc. will expose them to gluten through skin contact. I am happy to provide gluten-free substitutes for all of these materials or will call the manufacturer to verify gluten-free status of the products you now use.

The kids want to bring cold lunch most days this year. I will get the menu from the West Des Moines dietician office again this year and will mark the days and items they can eat on hot lunch days. For aftercare, they will need to get something from their snack box in the room if they can't eat what the other kids are having.

Please call me at anytime when you have questions or concerns. Both kids have adjusted well to the condition and how they need to manage it. They do well in an atmosphere of relaxed, knowledgeable, alert awareness of potentially unsafe conditions whenever food is available. I appreciate your providing the extra communication their special dietary needs require. It takes more time and I am very grateful for your efforts in both keeping Joe and Sam healthy and feeling included in the class activities.

Sincerely, ✍

Being A Teen With Celiac

As If Acne Wasn't Bad Enough

It's tough enough being a teen,
I think you know just what I mean.
But I won't let this diet,
Cause me to riot.
It's a challenge, but I'll stay serene.

Food For Thought
by Jonathan Borders

I was diagnosed with celiac disease in November 2002 at age 17. I had been experiencing many problems with my skin for two years, and it kept being misdiagnosed. Finally it was determined I had dermatitis herpetiformis, a skin disease commonly linked to celiac disease. I was tested for celiac disease and the results came back positive.

It has been a really big pain for me to find food to eat and it's very hard not to cheat, especially when I go out with friends. However, I have found my friends to be very supportive and often let me pick the restaurants where we eat. Many of my friends have even cooked food for me occasionally. It has been a pain getting used to saying "no" when people offer me pizza or a sandwich but it has now become a habit and I just have to keep in mind it is for the best.

Many times, I feel a sudden urge,
To say, "Screw this diet," and go on a
    splurge.
I simply want the opportunity to eat,
Something other than fruit, veggies,
    and meat.
I want to feel no guilt in my head,

For eating a slice of freshly baked bread.
I want to eat a bagel and some
cinnamon rolls,
Some warm glazed donuts and even
some donut holes.
It's really not too bad, constantly eating
steak,
But I would kill for an entire chocolate
cake.
Lord knows I'm not a big drinker of
booze,
But I'd like to know I could have some
if I choose.
I wanna go to Fazoli's and eat some
spaghetti,
And eat a pizza while watching Mario
Andretti.
I wanna be able to buy bread at Great
Harvest,
Of all of their loaves, I'd buy the very
largest.
For Thanksgiving, I want to eat some
pumpkin pie,
I'd eat a stack of pies as high as the sky.
I want chocolate chip cookies straight
out of the oven,
Washed down with some milk that
would give my stomach some lovin'.
I want some of my mom's homemade
lasagna,
I'd eat it so fast I might even get some on ya.

I wanna go to Panera and eat what I
    desire,
And cool down with a Klondike bar
    when I perspire.
I wanna eat the bread during
    communion time,
And to be true to Scripture, follow it
    down with some wine.
O Food, my Love, I feel so betrayed!!!
I feel like a dog that's just been neutered
    or spayed!
Lord, I can't wait for the banquet table
    in eternity,
When the food I eat won't have to be
    gluten-free.

Cold Days And Clear Skies

by Mandy Taylor

My name is Mandy and I'm 16 years old. I was diagnosed with celiac disease less than a year ago after having symptoms for about four years. I love playing soccer, hanging out with my friends, listening to Coldplay and Dave Matthews Band, and now, eating!

My eyes are shut tight. I'm relying on my senses of smell, taste, and touch to keep this piece of pizza real, just in case when I open my eyes it's not there. The crust is warm and moist in my hands. I can feel some rogue strands of cheese dangling over the edge, and droplets of grease and rich tomato sauce fall onto my hand. I open my eyes just for a split second, and the pepperoni seems to smile at me, just waiting for me to enjoy this delicacy. I close my eyes again and slowly start to bring this slice of pizza toward my mouth, which is already watering at the thought of this culinary delight coming in contact with my taste buds, "Mandy!"

My eyes fly open and I'm face to face with a friend of mine, who's just exited the lunch line. I guiltily hand over her pizza, which I was holding while she purchased a carton of milk and three luscious looking chocolate chip cookies. My daydream is shattered, and I'm back in the real world, the world of rice pasta, corn flour, and of course, pieces of pizza that beckon unfairly. However, I'm not disappointed. The daydream will be back

I have the honor of having an immune system that amuses itself by pretending gluten is poison, and intestines that, apparently bored of their mundane life, go along with the joke.

again. Until then, I have a delicious chocolate fudge brownie to enjoy, made, of course, with the "oh so decadent" rice flour.

I may be only 16 years old, and barely starting to make any sort of distinguishable impact on the world around me, but I am already one of the most unique people at my high school. I have the honor of having an immune system that amuses itself by pretending gluten is poison, and intestines that, apparently bored of their mundane life, go along with the joke. Yes, I am a celiac, a proud member of the exclusive club of funky immune systems. A part of me still thinks this is a pretty unfair deal. The same part of me that wants to scream like a maniac as I watch my friends eat. But another part of me, the rational part, thinks that along with my disease, I am pretty unique. And so is my story.

I experienced the first of what I call celiac attacks when I was 12. That incident seems to have blocked itself from my memory, but I do recall a night during my family's vacation in Hawaii. I don't remember what I ate, but I remember the worst stomach pain I have ever had, and being in the bathroom all night. My memory then flashes forward two years to a soccer practice with my club team. Running along in a scrimmage, I was suddenly stricken with the most intense stomach pain. My brain couldn't even seem to comprehend this pain as I lay on the grass dizzy and in a fog. On the way home I brilliantly ate a chicken quesadilla on, of course, a flour tortilla. When I returned home, it was all I could do to writhe on my bed. My 14-year-old brain figured this sort of pain must be death. Sitting up on my bed, my room began to spin in fast circles, and I passed out on my floor. Upon waking up, sweaty, the pain was gone, and there was a buzzing in my ears so loud it sounded like there was a bee hive hidden in my shirt. I don't remember telling my parents what happened. All I know is soon I was in the emergency room, being told the pain was simply that time of the month that every girl has to endure. I figured these doctors knew what they were talking about, and I let it go.

This horrible experience left a huge impression on me, and I would never forget that pain. I only prayed it wouldn't happen again. But it did. It happened again, and again, and again, until I was afraid to eat anything, afraid to leave the house, afraid to live my life. Each time the waves of pain and dizziness swept over me, I only wanted it to kill me. It seemed to be the only thing to make the pain stop. And each time I woke up from passing out, whether it was lying shivering in the bathroom or huddled in the hallway, the hopelessness I felt was nearly as unbearable as the pain

An entire year of having these attacks slowly went by. When I was 15, I underwent arthroscopic surgery on my right knee, as a result of chronic pain that had mysteriously developed. The surgeon discovered numerous cracks on the underside of my kneecap. I didn't know it then, but this too was a result of this disease that was ravaging my body. Along with the knee problem and the stomach pain attacks, I experienced bad headaches almost daily. I had trouble sleeping and focusing on school. My stomach was so bloated that I sometimes appeared pregnant. My vision deteriorated as well. When I was 13, I had been told I was legally blind in my left eye, and over a year later my once perfect right eye vision rapidly began to join my left. Whatever illness I had, it was taking over my life. I began to lose touch with my best friends because I was always sick. Some days I would simply go without eating. During one particular severe episode after my knee operation, I lost 11 pounds in a week from living off a bowl of applesauce a day. I needed answers, and fast.

I began to see doctor after doctor. My childhood doctor, having known me since babyhood, figured because I had nearly always been a little sickly (I suffered from sinus infections from infancy on), that this was just another one of those times. I saw her at least four times, and she told me each time my problem was bad cramps and a sensitive stomach. The

Several months were spent deeply depressed, thinking that my life was over. I couldn't be around my friends because I couldn't stop thinking they could eat whatever they wanted.

doctors at the emergency room also thought it was cramps, and perhaps a little anxiety. After countless blood, stool, and urine tests that seemed to find nothing, I was told I would grow out of it. Everyone else seemed to think I was a hypochondriac, and my hope was fading fast.

One afternoon, while surfing the Internet looking for illnesses with my symptoms, I found a medical posting Web site. Pure impulse made me post my symptoms on that Web site, sparking what tiny shreds of hope for a diagnosis I had left. Over the next few days, I read the answers to my post, which told me it sounded like I had irritable bowel syndrome. I was elated, thrilled that I was finally getting some sort of answer. After spending days reading about this syndrome, I received an e-mail from someone at the posting site. The e-mail told me it may very well be irritable bowel syndrome. However, had I heard of celiac disease?

My mom made countless urgent phone calls to my doctor, who finally made an appointment for me with a gastroenterologist. The day I walked into this doctor's office was the day that changed me. Right away he seemed to recognize my symptoms as celiac disease and wanted to get a definite diagnosis right away. Although this would involve a colonoscopy, not the friendliest of procedures, and small bowel biopsy, I was elated. I could have a diagnosis!

I spent a weekend prepping for the procedures: two fun-filled days of strong laxatives and clear liquids. It would have gotten a little boring, but luckily I had stocked the bathroom with a good supply of magazines. Another day was spent at the hospital, having a tube shoved down one end and up another. Not fun at the time, but now I look back and realize it was a little amusing. It was all worth it a week later, when we got a call from the doctor. My diagnosis: a severe case of celiac sprue. And so began my life.

Something important has been taken from us for reasons we're not sure about, whether it's our genes or just bad luck. We must learn to fill that hole with whatever we can.

It took several months for the fact to sink in that I could no longer have wheat, oats, rye, malt, and barley, which, of course, are included in seemingly every food, beverage, and sauce on this planet. I felt even sorrier for myself than I had when I was still very sick. It made me want to cry when I looked at pizza or cake, or walked into the mall and smelled the aroma of the world's best cinnamon rolls. Several months were spent deeply depressed, thinking that my life was over. I couldn't be around my friends because I couldn't stop thinking they could eat whatever they wanted. When I was around them, I blew up at them countless times for enjoying their cookies or pasta or numerous other things. Days were spent staring longingly at the box of fettuccine alfredo in our cupboard and at the package of chocolate muffins on top of the refrigerator. I stifled so many urges to stuff as many hot dog buns in my mouth as I could. But as the long days passed, something changed. I went a full month without a severe attack. I began to sleep better. I was learning, and along with the learning came living.

My mom and I began to enjoy experimenting with different recipes. We mostly made brownies, trying nearly every gluten-free recipe we could find, and then gorging ourselves on them afterward. One evening, for the first time in months, I enjoyed a delicious plate of rich cheese fettuccine, made with the rice pasta I had mistakenly thought would be disgusting. The pasta was, instead, even better than "normal" pasta. So were the brownies. Pretty soon, so was the cake. And then so was the pizza.

Something changed in those days of experimenting and shopping and making discoveries. It was me. Slowly, my view on life began to change. Yes, I had a disease, and yes, it was a very serious one, but there was no way it was going to stop me from enjoying the life I finally had back. I began enjoying the little things again, something years before I had prided myself on.

I had a few laughs as my friends tried to digest my diagnosis, constantly saying things like, "But…pasta doesn't have wheat in it, right?" and, "Well, at least you can have potato bread, since it's made out of potatoes." I even heard a few, "Ohh, I know exactly how you feel. I'm on a diet, too." But gradually the confusion gave way to understanding, and they supported me. So did my parents. My dad, by making constant runs to the store to pick up something I was craving, and my mom, by spending 24 hours in the kitchen concocting all sorts of meals which always turned out to be surprisingly delicious.

My energy came back, and so did my love for life. My headaches subsided, and my stomach bloat began to look only two months pregnant instead of six or seven. After my last surgical procedure (a laparoscopy to check and see if any of my other organs were scarred) was finally over, my junior year in high school began. It was a new beginning after a horrific summer of pain, surgery, and hopelessness. I played on my school's varsity soccer team, and began to fully enjoy school again. I was finally healthy and planned on staying that way. I knew because of my entire ordeal, I would never even consider drinking, smoking, or drugs. It had taken so much effort and energy to regain my health, I would do nothing to ruin it.

One afternoon, I sat at my desk at home studying for a math test and craving about a thousand different foods. As I began to feel slowly overwhelmed, I heard a rumbling outside and looked up to see the UPS truck pull up our driveway. It was the gluten-free donuts and hot dog buns I had ordered from a wonderful gluten-free food company. I tore open the box and took my first bite of a rich chocolate donut. It was the smallest thing for most people; a bite of a donut, but the second it took me to take that bite simply made my day.

It's the little things like that we celiacs must remember to enjoy. Something important has been taken from us for reasons we're not sure about, whether it's our genes or just bad luck. We must learn to fill that hole with whatever we can. In a way, we are all blessed. Yeah, this disease isn't fun, but even though it's taken many things from my life, it's given me so much more. I love everything about life now. I love being with my amazing friends and family. I love cold days and clear skies. I love when I look at the car across from me on the road and see the person inside singing along to the same song on the radio I'm listening to. I love putting on clothes warm from the dryer. I love when friends hug me good morning. And, I love it when my cat falls off a chair and tries to pretend she meant to all along. In short, I love the little things. I realize life is not all about everything being perfect. It's just about enjoying what you have. And I have celiac disease to thank for that. I could have been handed a disease that would end my life. Instead, I was lucky enough to have a disease that would help it to begin again.

When You're A Teen

by Jennifer Griffin

I am a 21-year-old from Stony Point, New York. I first learned I had celiac disease as a 16-year-old. Presently I am a senior at Bucknell University and am planning to pursue a Master's Degree in Social Work. I hope to someday be a private therapist working with adolescents.

Shortly after celebrating my sweet sixteen, I was diagnosed with celiac disease. At first, I was so relieved the doctors found out what was wrong with me. After months of feeling sick, the doctors finally knew what I was suffering from. To be honest with you, I was so happy because they were actually going to take me seriously, after months of telling me nothing was wrong. I had no idea, though, of the long road to recovery that was ahead of me.

When my doctor told me I had celiac disease, he didn't tell me of the feelings of isolation I would have following the diagnosis. I think these feelings were intensified because of my age. As a teenage celiac, I often felt out of the loop. The trips to McDonald's and the high school cafeteria often reminded me I was "different" than most teenagers, and left my mouth watering. The strange looks I received when a waiter put a salad down on my plate, and the rest of my friends were eating hamburgers and fries, hurt my feelings.

When I began my college search, celiac disease was becoming a larger part of my life, if you can even imagine that being possible. When I was looking into schools it was apparent I was different than other high school juniors. Most teenagers ask about the social life when they visit college campuses. Not me. I asked if on campus apartments were available.

Shortly after being diagnosed, I came to realize a celiac has to be assertive. When you go to a restaurant, you have to make sure the cook knows what gluten is. Being a teenager, it's often difficult to get people to take you seriously. I have often received nasty looks when I insisted the hamburger shouldn't touch the hamburger bun. What the waitress or waiter doesn't understand is I'm not being difficult, I'm just keeping myself from becoming sick.

If you're a teenager, I think having a teenage support group can be extremely beneficial. It's good to have people your own age to talk to about the feelings you're having and certain circumstances you're experiencing. You can share and learn a lot of helpful tips that would be useful in our lifestyle. Personally, I would have loved to hear some advice from people my own age about how to make the feelings of isolation less severe. ✍

Jennifer's mother, Donna, has written "Celiac Disease 101," which can be read in Chapter 12 and "Doing Disney Gluten-Free," which can be read in Chapter 10.

Mixed Feelings

by Alexa Gordon

My name is Alexa Gordon. I am a 13-year-old girl who was diagnosed a year-and-a-half ago with celiac disease. Now I am more accustomed to having celiac and I'm living a wonderful gluten-free life with my parents and sister, Carolyn, 11. Celiac is a challenge, and I'm glad I am still living a happy and HEALTHY life!

All my life I was smaller than most people. Everyone around me knew it and some even joked about it. Not only was I shorter than almost everyone in my grade, but even my younger sister had outgrown me. My family has never been the tallest of people, but even by their standards, I was small, both in height and weight. The older I got the further behind I fell.

My name is Alexa Gordon. I am now almost 13 years old and was diagnosed with celiac only about a year-and-a-half ago. Looking back, I can't truthfully say it was one of the easier things in life to deal with emotionally. In fact, there were MANY times when I felt like it was the most awful thing in the world.

For years I had frequent stomach aches, but few other symptoms to make it clear what was wrong with me. So, every doctor I went to simply said I was eating things that didn't agree with me and would probably be petite when I grew up.

Then, about two years ago, I went with my parents to see a gastroenterologist at Children's Hospital of Philadelphia. The doctor listened while my mom described my symptoms and explained why it worried her and my dad. The doctor asked my mother about her ethnic background and also my father's. When my mom explained she is Italian and my father is mostly Scottish and Irish, the doctor immediately asked if I had been tested for celiac. It turns out this disease is common among those ethnic groups. My parents were very relieved that we might finally know what was wrong with me.

I had mixed feelings. I was glad we might have found the cause of my stomach aches and growth problems, but I was scared I might have a "disease." My parents told me I had to have a surgical procedure to prove I had celiac. I began to cry, afraid of having to be put to sleep while a camera tube was put down my throat to see my stomach.

The good news: The procedure wasn't as bad as I had feared.

The bad news: The test proved I had celiac.

I now had to go on a very strict diet. If I were to make any error in what I ate, I could become very sick and possibly cause myself permanent growth problems.

It quickly got annoying, having to look at every food label to see if ANY ingredient had even a trace of gluten. The problem was, I was just starting with this new "diet" and I didn't know which ingredients had gluten and which didn't. My mom helped me a lot by researching all ingredients derived from wheat, barley, oats, and rye. We even had to research ingredients the manufacturers weren't sure about.

We went to a nutritionist to see if I could catch up to where my height and weight should have been if I didn't have celiac disease. To help me catch up, I had to take four to five pills a day and a 300 calorie supplement twice a day. It became very difficult. I started feeling really down all the time and was not acting at all like my usual self. I went into a rut for at least six months and often felt sad.

My family was concerned and asked me what was wrong, but I didn't know. This made me confused and sadder. I felt as if I was never happy and many of my loved ones probably thought the same thing about me.

Slowly I began to become used to having this disease 24/7. I started hanging out more with my friends and doing more things that a normal girl my age would do. I just had to realize I was not weird, and that made me feel a little better. What really did it for me was KNOWING and BELIEVING that even though I had been through all those challenges and troubles, I still had made it. I knew I would never really be the same as I used to be before knowing about my celiac disease, but I felt like I was a much stronger person and I still do. I had dealt with the, "Why aren't you eating that" and, "What is gluten?" questions, and even some of the unavoidable, "Ew, that's gross," comments about my unusual, gluten-free food. I had learned from these experiences how much people's words can have a negative effect on others.

One of the worst feelings I have experienced as a person with celiac disease is when I'm with everyone else at a party and I stick out like a sore thumb because I can't have the pizza! "That stupid pizza," I used to think. But it wasn't the pizza that made me feel bad. It was all the people around me.

They looked at me funny because I wasn't eating 'normal' food. I just wanted to go home because I didn't want to stick out like that. I wanted to blend in and just, for once, be NORMAL!

Now, after my many experiences in these situations, I think being normal is highly overrated, and that it's better to be unique. If you are different, be proud and don't be a "normal wannabe" like I used to be. If you offered anyone with celiac disease the chance to get rid of it forever, they would probably do it in a heartbeat, right? Maybe you too, but not me.

I think having celiac has been the biggest learning experience of my life and I would love to someday have the chance to help find a cure. Until then, all I can do is hope that sharing my experience will help others.

The truth is, no one but you knows how bad your celiac can be. Well intentioned people might say they "understand," but to really understand they'd have to be YOU. Anyone can say you're "weird" because you have a disease, but there are SO many other people out there who have diseases, many of which are worse than celiac. I feel there are so many other people out there "fighting" a disease, but we are special, because we are overcoming celiac disease by living with it, each day.

Knowing that helps us hold our heads high everyday. ✍

Gluten-Free Tears

by Claire Poppe

I was diagnosed with celiac disease more than five years ago. It was before my sophomore year of high school, after a freshman year consisting of gastrointestinal pain and severe anemia. I feel blessed the diagnosis only took a year to make! I plan to go to graduate school for chemistry after traveling abroad in Germany.

I would like to thank my family for all of their love and support (both culinary and emotional). I couldn't have managed without it!

This was written two-and-a-half years after my diagnosis as part of my senior English project on "The Meaning of Life." This poem no longer reflects my true feelings. In the past three years I have gotten over my bitterness and have learned to go with the flow. Yes, it has taken time and adjustment, oh do I ever know. Poetry has been, and remains, a way for me to work through my frustrations. It helps when you just want to scream.

gluten-free tears
microbial molecular happenings:
my downfall
rubbing,
disintegrating,
eroding like the intestinal Mississippi
chunks of fleshy absorption whittled
     away by that monstrosity
plagues my existence.
really not an issue
pizza smells better by far than it ever
     tasted, right?
right, mom?
mom?
cannot tell a lie – further repercussions
     of damn glorified cherry tree
at least I can eat cherries
no normal pie for me
though I'm "special"
so many kids long to be special
well, at times it sucks
so eat your fresh, warm, crusty bread
and let me weep
wallow in self-pity
it does a girl good once in a while
a long while.

Not Bad, An Inconvenience

by Stephanie Campbell

My name is Stephanie and I grew up and live in Colorado. I am 16 years old and a sophomore in high school. I love to play sports and hang out with my friends. We even eat out together and my celiac has not stopped me yet. My favorite activities are wood working and playing the piano. I also have two dogs whom I love and a very supportive family.

I will not say it is bad to have celiac disease. Instead, I will say it is an inconvenience you must get used to. I am currently able to eat gluten-free pizzas and great spaghetti. Even though I have celiac disease, I live a pretty normal life.

I am 16 and can remember how a year ago I was dealing with unbelievable pain in my stomach. The pain was so bad I was hospitalized twice. Despite many tests: a CAT scan, ultrasound, and a host of others, no one could figure out what was wrong. Finally, one day after I had come home from school, my mom told me the doctor called and said I had gluten intolerance.

I immediately went to the computer and looked it up on the Internet. I went to various Web sites, celiac.com and webmd.com, to find out what gluten intolerance was and what I had to do to treat it. I soon found out what I could and could not eat. Some things were obvious such as wheat and oats. Other things were surprising such as licorice and soy sauce.

As if it wasn't stressful enough having to rearrange my diet, I was losing weight because of the disease's effect on my digestive system. There was also added stress because I had to deal with my new diet in school. It wasn't as difficult as I thought to get my teachers to allow me to eat in their classes if necessary. I simply explained I had a wheat allergy and may need to eat food in their classrooms. They were very nice about it and even concerned.

It turned out to be a lot harder dealing with my friends. They felt sorry for me and they just didn't understand what I was going through. I found, however, the more I educated them on my condition and told them how I was feeling, the more they understood about my adjustments, emotionally and physically. It was frustrating and difficult to hear them say they were sorry and concerned while knowing they hardly understood what was really happening. I didn't blame them. I had to figure out how to help them identify with what was happening to me, the pain I was in, and the difficulty I had. That made it easier for them to comprehend what I was going through.

It's been a challenging year but I am happy to say things are going well. I'm feeling a whole lot better. My family and I have used cookbooks to help us enjoy delicious family meals. It has been a year since my diagnosis and one of my friends even went to the trouble to bake a gluten-free cake for his birthday so I could participate in the celebration.

Best of luck to everyone affected by celiac or know someone who is.

Senior Celiacs

Ain't No Stopping Me Now

> *As I grow older things become clear,*
> *And my health becomes very dear.*
> *If I eat what I should,*
> *One thing's understood.*
> *Celiac, I won't have to fear.*

When You're A Little "Older"

by Diana Marks

My husband was diagnosed with celiac disease when he was 59. At that time we had been married for 25 years. Adjusting our lives in our advancing years was quite a challenge. We however learned that "you can teach an old dog new tricks."

O ur family has been living with celiac disease for about five years now. I thought I would share some tips for living with the disease when you're a little "older" (we're in our fifties).

Hospital Stays:
Being that we're in our "advanced" years we tend to have more things go wrong and hospital stays become something you have to deal with. Believe it or not, many dietary problems are created when a celiac has to be a patient in a hospital. If you are hospitalized, please do not assume the correct food will be delivered on your tray just because you're in the hospital. During my husband's first hospital stay after being diagnosed with celiac disease, we carefully made arrangements with the hospital dietician informing her about his special needs. Unfortunately items containing gluten were

served with his meals. This can be a big problem, especially if the patient is a bit groggy and no one is there to monitor the delivered tray. Bring in some food from home so if you're served something you can't eat, you won't go hungry. It's also very important to find an advocate to do the monitoring for you.

Airline Travel:

Now that we've reached our golden years and the kids are out of the house it's a perfect time to do some traveling. We decided not to let celiac disease get in the way. I would not expend a lot of energy and time trying to get the airlines (if food is served) to provide gluten-free meals. Just be prepared to take your own food on the trip. With airline travel as it is now, special meals often do not arrive as ordered and frequently airline flights are cancelled or changed. Little cans of tuna, fruit, nuts, gluten-free crackers, and small juice boxes are easy to pack. Now you don't have to worry about airline cooperation.

Trips:

We have found some groups that put together trips and cruises especially for celiacs. They make all the arrangements and find restaurants wherever the trip takes you. We have had very good times and met very nice people.

Cruises:

We have been on several cruises. If you make arrangements beforehand, and then double check them when you get on board, you should be very pleased. Each night my husband was given a special menu to decide what he wanted for his meals the next day. They have been very accommodating and we have had some great times. There was always plenty of fruit on board and my husband has never gone hungry.

I guess the moral of my celiac story is: your life doesn't have to be different from everyone else's, just your food has to be. ✍🏻

Adjusting At 55

by Myra Lee

My husband and I have been married for 35 years. We have two adult children who, fortunately, are not celiacs. Since my husband was diagnosed with celiac in his late fifties we had to learn how to adjust our lives at a time when adjusting isn't always that easy.

My husband was diagnosed with celiac disease in his late fifties. He was always healthy and was even still playing tennis. One day he began to feel very sick to his stomach. Nothing would stay down, or in him. At first the doctors thought he had a bad stomach virus. After he lost 20 pounds and could barely function, they began to think it must be more serious. He began a series of many tests ("oscopy" this and "oscopy" that). The doctors could find no reason for him to be as sick as he was. One doctor even wanted to do exploratory surgery!

We decided to go out of our health network and visit a famous hospital. After more tests, one doctor finally thought my husband had celiac disease and put him on a gluten-free diet. It was a miracle! He instantly felt better and even began to gain some weight. He didn't even need medication.

That was the good news. The bad news is he has a condition which he will have for the rest of his life. After being used to eating anything and anywhere he wanted, now his diet would have to be strictly managed.

The first thing the doctors suggested was to visit a nutritionist. We discovered most nutritionists are not well informed since ours told us you only have to be concerned with the first five ingredients on a label. A big buzzer went off in our heads since by this time we, luckily, had done enough research to know this was incorrect information.

We found the best sources of information about managing the disease are from other people who are celiacs and who live the diet. There are also many helpful Web sites on the Internet. Of course every celiac has to remember they must be responsible for themselves. You have to verify the safety of the products you choose to use and the restaurants you choose to visit.

We now know that everyone has to find their own way to manage their diet. Different people have different sensitivities and tolerances. The key to the diet is to figure out what you miss the most (in our case it was bagels and sandwich bread) and to set out to find acceptable alternatives so you do not feel so deprived. There are numerous gluten-free products on the market now and it becomes a question of taste and accessibility. Also, a positive attitude makes all the difference in the world.

Celiac, Traveling, And Osteoporosis

by Sandra Clayton

I was diagnosed with celiac disease in July 2003 at the age of 65. I am a retired nurse and have two children and four grandchildren. My son, two of my grandchildren, and my daughter-in-law all have celiac disease.

Before I was diagnosed with celiac disease in July 2003, my daughter-in-law, grandson, and granddaughter all had positive blood tests for celiac disease. My daughter-in-law felt I had a lot of celiac symptoms such as osteoporosis, lactose intolerance, and inability to gain weight (I weighed 108 pounds from 1960 through 2003!). To satisfy her continued urging, my son and I were tested. I never dreamed my test would come back positive. A few days before I received my results, my son was told he was positive. Then my results came in. Not only did I test positive but I had the dubious distinction of having the highest test results in the family!

I left the doctor's office, where I received no support or direction and went right to our local health store right here in

Mississauga, Ontario, Canada. I was given a tour of their gluten-free products and a list of them. I was able to buy raisin bread, a multi-grain loaf, carrot muffins, and a blueberry pie. Hey this wasn't going to be so bad! Thanks to my daughter-in-law, who had thoroughly researched the disease, I knew a lot about celiac. She also knew the headquarters for the Canadian Celiac Association was in Mississauga, which happens to be within two miles of my home. They were very helpful and gave me a book listing products I could still eat. My son and his family were wishing they still lived in Ontario instead of Phoenix, Arizona!

This diagnosis came right before I was scheduled to go on a 26 day bus tour through Great Britain and Ireland. I did not want to miss that. My sympathetic tour agent (her mom had the disease) was helpful and informed British Airways and the tour company. I took six packages of cookies and four packages of crackers and health bars. While I traveled, I kept baggies of these in my carry-on. Each hotel had been informed of my diet. Breakfasts were easy as they were all buffet style and I ate lots of different fruit and bacon. There was usually a bowl of fresh fruit and sometimes dried fruit or raisins which were great for mid-morning snacks. Lunches were more difficult, but my new friends and I read the menus before we went into the restaurant. I also discovered health stores where I was able to buy bread. I now had a slice at breakfast and carried two slices with me in case I needed them for lunch. I found a fantastic chain in some cities that carried raisin, lemon and fruit loaf cakes and fantastic coconut macaroons. I also stopped to buy fruit frequently as others on the trip did. Dinners were quite often buffet style so they were no problem and if it was a special outing it was fairly easy to adapt something on the menu. People at the food establishments were always very helpful. I was amazed at how easy the food was on the trip, but I am glad I brought snacks with me. I would certainly not hesitate to go traveling again.

I was shocked when I returned home to find I weighed 118 pounds. I even jumped off the scales and tried again. I knew I would gain weight on the diet if it was working, but I had never weighed that much except when I was pregnant.

I am lazy and live alone so I can afford to buy ready made gluten-free food. I have tried ten different types of bread and liked them all. I have cut out the cookies and pies in hopes of being able to still wear my clothes.

Having osteoporosis has been a big concern of mine since I was diagnosed at 52 years of age (I am 65 now). The doctor who tested me is a well known gynecologist and so is the geriatric specialist who treats my osteoporosis. But they never put together my symptoms to come up with the possible diagnosis of celiac disease. I would recommend anyone with osteoporosis be tested for celiac disease. It is now good to know that dietary changes can help reverse this condition and certainly keep the calcium depletion from getting worse.

I am so grateful that my son and grandchildren have been diagnosed at younger ages. Hopefully they will be spared some of the bone loss that I experienced.

Sandra's daughter-in-law, Sue, has written "Living With Celiac Disease: Our First Year," and her granddaughter, Angie, has written "My First Gluten-Free Halloween," both of which can be read in Chapter Three. Her grandson, Kevin, has written "Who Wants A Cookie," which can be read in Chapter Four.

I'm Going To Dinner

by Welda Clemens

I was born and raised in Escondido, California, and have dealt with the symptoms of celiac disease since the age of eight. An elementary school teacher for 25 years, I retired in 2002 and opened an Indian arts gift shop named Felicita's Place. I have three grown children and seven grandchildren and am currently taking care of my newest grandson, eight-month-old Dakota. Dakota was diagnosed two months ago with gluten sensitivity and allergies to milk and dairy. I've written several books on San Diego County Indian history and continue to research that subject, as well as the subject of celiac disease.

I'm going to dinner with my best friend tonight. We're both 59 and enjoy sharing birthday dinners with my sister, who is one year older. However, I always seem to stress out about, "What will I eat?" since I have celiac disease. In addition to being allergic to wheat and all grains, I am also allergic to all milk and dairy products, as well as egg whites and yeast. I've had asthma since the age of eight and I used to feel so sorry for myself, because when I ate certain foods I would tighten up, wheeze profusely and be unable to breathe. The doctors told me that if I didn't go for allergy testing by the age of 19, I would be bedridden by the age of

25. Since I already had two babies I certainly wanted to be well.

After all the tests and three years of shots, I was still suffering the same fate. Nothing seemed to help, although when I would fast I would always be able to breathe better. Finally, in my 30's, I began eliminating wheat and milk, since those always caused me to wheeze. Over 20 years later I was told, while having a colonoscopy, I had celiac disease. I had always known there was a name for what was ailing me.

That was two years ago and was when I first connected with the celiac Web site. I was surprised to learn that so many people in America and throughout the world have this same disease. Recently my newborn grandson exhibited signs of milk allergy, so I sent away for a home test, only to learn that he is gluten intolerant and allergic to all milk and dairy. That is spurring me on to develop new recipes and to learn more effective ways of helping family members realize what a serious disease this is.

My father died of colon cancer, and I suspect that is where our celiac originates, so I am adamant about working to get other family members tested too. We have attention deficit disorder, food allergies, sinus problems, migraines, thyroid cancer, hepatitis C, diabetes, and other serious ailments as part of our family history.

I am hoping others will do whatever is necessary to learn what is causing their distress, then move to make changes. I have never felt better. I think I'll pack a bag to take along to dinner tonight, just in case the restaurant's offerings are limited. I've learned to do that, and to take good care of myself so I will be around to help take care of my family!

Finally At 67

by Shirley Whitley

I was born in Indiana in 1934. Since age nine I have had many undiagnosed health problems. It took until age 67 to finally get a diagnosis of celiac disease. I have been gluten-free since my biopsy, but have developed many problems probably because of the length of time it took me to be diagnosed.

In 1940, my parents emigrated from Indiana to Arizona because of my mother's severe asthma, not to mention her digestive problems. I was then about six-and-a-half years old. When I was nine I began to develop severe allergies, mostly to pollens.

At age 13, I developed a severe rash on my lower legs. When my doctor could not solve the problem he referred us to an allergist and a dermatologist. These doctors tested me for everything and one thing I tested allergic to was wheat. They took me off wheat for three weeks, (which was not long enough) but the rash didn't go away. Since I did not respond, they put me back on wheat because "I was so painfully thin."

They experimented with me for three years and finally told my mother to take me to a psychiatrist because this weepy, itchy, sticky rash I had was obviously in my head.

Finally my family practice doctor suggested the ocean to help heal the rash. In 1950, my parents took me to San Diego for a month. The ocean did heal the rash, at least temporarily, and we went back to Phoenix.

In college the rash returned with a vengeance and we went back to San Diego where I met my soon-to-be husband. We married six months later.

Flashing forward about 15 years, I began developing bouts of severe alternating diarrhea and constipation. I was also feeling extremely tired all of the time. This went on until I was 67 years old.

As luck would have it I, along with most of the family, came down with a case of intestinal flu from my grandchildren. Everyone else in the family got over it but I did not. It was so bad I could not leave the house for six weeks, lost 35 pounds, and could barely walk. One day I was watching television and I saw Danna Korn and her son talking about celiac disease. Since I had a doctor's appointment the next day, I went and requested a celiac panel. The doctor was reluctant to order it because I was somewhat overweight and "just could not have celiac disease." I insisted and he gave me the test. Two weeks later he called to tell me I tested very positive and he referred me to a gastroenterologist who confirmed my diagnosis with a biopsy.

I have developed multiple problems because of this late diagnosis: a severely compromised immune system, multiple allergies, joint pain, and extreme fatigue. For anyone out there, if your family has a history of gastric or skin problems that are undiagnosed, please, please consider celiac disease and try to convince your doctor to give you the tests.

Success With Celiac

You Don't Have To Be A Gluten For Punishment

> *Some restaurants thought I was weird,*
> *When I told them the foods that I feared.*
> *But now they're okay,*
> *With my celiac way.*
> *As a customer I'm highly revered.*

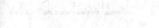

My First Big Challenge: Eating Out

by Sandy Adams

Having lived in the beautiful Northwest for many years, I love the outdoors and gardening. Pottery is my passion and teaching was my vocation. I share my home with five parrots and three pomeranians. It has been five years since I found I had celiac disease and it took a while to determine what was causing nausea and skin rashes. Celiac disease has changed what I eat but not my life.

Being a celiac, having a tendency toward high cholesterol and also being a vegetarian has significantly lessened my choices of food. However, at home, I eat a diet of things I really enjoy and have been able to maintain my weight and health as well. My first big challenge was eating out with friends and also going to people's houses for dinner. These are the ways I've learned to deal with different situations:

1) I always try to get familiar with the menus at restaurants before I go. That way I don't have to quiz or put the waiter on the spot and make an issue in front of my friends.

2) When invited to a friend's home I always ask if I can bring something and of course, it is always something I can eat.

3) I eat something at home before I go. My friends have been very good about often catering to my diet, but it makes me somewhat uncomfortable for them to do that. I don't want them to limit what they want to serve.

4) The important thing is being with friends and not the food. People don't understand the consequences of breaking a diet for a celiac and I dislike having to explain it all the time.

It works for me. I hope it helps you.

A View From College

by Joshua Marks

I am originally from the Chicago area and have lived in New York City for nine years where I taught Special Education and Social Studies at a public high school. Currently I am in Chiang Mai, Thailand, taking a one year leave of absence. This piece was written when I was a junior in college.

I would like to thank Sue Goldstein and Leslie Elsner for "saving my life." If not for them I would still be walking around grocery store aisles in circles.

When I was diagnosed with celiac disease I did not understand exactly what I was up against. The doctor made it sound as if it was no big deal. I was told, like so many other celiacs, "Oh, you just have to eliminate gluten from your diet." However, I soon realized there was a lot more to it than that.

I had just turned 21 when I found out I had celiac disease. It was the beginning of my sophomore year and as most college students do, I lived on pizza, bagels, muffins, and sandwiches. I also frequently attended a number of parties where I enjoyed beer and grain alcohol. I didn't yet realize the extent to which I had to change my life. Once I found out just about everything I ate contained gluten, I knew I needed to make some major adjustments.

The major adjustment I faced was dealing with social situations. At parties and formal dinners, I found there was nothing I could eat and no alcohol I could drink. My mother didn't have too much sympathy for my inability to digest alcohol, but most college students will tell you drinking is a major part of college life. I felt very awkward at parties explaining why I had to turn down a beer. I became very self conscious and as a result, I rarely attended any social gatherings. When going to a restaurant on a date I hated explaining why I couldn't order anything from the menu. I felt so bad, that I barely went out at all. In addition, before my disease, I was accustomed to grabbing a bagel or slice of pizza between classes. However, after I was diagnosed I wasn't able to do that anymore. In fact, I would not eat anything all day and just wait until I returned to my apartment to broil a chicken breast.

My not eating and self-pity lifestyle made things in school much worse. I would get annoyed and irritated by people and events that never bothered me before.

This routine of starving myself all day and not going out lasted about two depressing months. My not eating and self-pity lifestyle made things in school much worse. I would get annoyed and irritated by people and events that never bothered me before. I became very short tempered and didn't want to deal with anything or anybody. My grades and class work were affected. Every time I sat down to study, all I could think about was how angry I felt. I even stopped attending class because I couldn't learn anything. The only thing that entered my mind was how hungry I was and the foods I could not eat. It was definitely no way to live and required a change.

When I was close to going insane, I was forced to make a decision. I could let this lifelong disease control me or I could get my act together and control my disease. I decided to get my act together and kick my disease's butt. Before my diagnosis, the only cooking I ever did was making eggs on Sunday mornings. Now I had to learn how to cook food I could eat. Actually, this turned out to be easier than I thought. Also, I would prepare gluten-free sandwiches and bring them with me to school. When I went to restaurants I boldly brought my own bread and cookies. My attendance at social functions increased and I even found several items I could eat or drink. Sometimes I would even bring my own potato vodka and

When I start getting down about my disease, I try and concentrate on the good aspects of my life and, thank God, there are a lot of them.

share it with everyone. If a lot of my friends were going out, I would eat something at home first to reduce my hunger. Then, with my friends, I would order something simple like fries or potato skins after checking to be sure there was no cross-contamination in the frying oil from breaded items. My situation started to get a lot better.

As a result of my new control over my disease I became much more confident. I didn't mind answering questions like, "You can't have bread! What can you possibly eat?" I learned to laugh at these questions and give a friendly reply. Now, when I am faced with questions about my disease, I answer them and change the subject. I don't insist on explaining how difficult it is and how lucky everyone else is that they can eat all kinds of good foods.

This disease affects a person's everyday life. No one realizes the role food plays in his or her life until it is taken away. I could let myself get depressed over the situation or I could accept it and think about other aspects in my life. I decided a long time ago in order for me to be happy, I need to face my circumstances with a positive attitude. When I start getting down about my disease, I try and concentrate on the good aspects of my life and, thank God, there are a lot of them. If I focus too much on my disease it will pollute my life and make me a bitter person instead of a better person. I definitely don't want that to happen.

Adjusting has been and still is very difficult. Fortunately, as my everyday routine continues, things get much easier. Recently I have stopped desiring food I used to enjoy. Bakery goods never enter my mind. Even pizza doesn't seem so good anymore. Occasionally I get frustrated and annoyed. When that happens I just think that I am a normal human being who has been dealt a certain hand and I am living with it. Actually, if I may say so, I am doing a damn good job.

My good friends know I can't have certain foods so they have stopped offering them to me. Sometimes they even look out for my diet restrictions which I take as a sign they care. Now when I go out on a date or even with some friends, I find it to be no big deal to explain what I can't eat. Actually I turn things around and emphasize the food I can eat. I make my situation sound positive which makes everyone, including myself, feel more comfortable. That is the most important for me, to be at ease with my situation.

A year ago when I was diagnosed, I never imagined that I could be handling things the way I do. I even realized some positive things about my situation. Becoming a celiac made me more aware of nutrition. Ironically my disease has made me become a healthier person. I feel a hundred times better than I have in the past four years. I was able to cure myself from constant episodes of pain and fatigue and replace them with humor and rice crackers. I know what I can and can't have and because of it I feel great. I love living without pain and I have so much energy I sometimes don't know what to do with all of it. The way I see it, celiac disease all depends on how a person decides to live with it. I am able to view it on a positive note only because I chose to control it rather than letting it control me. I can't imagine living any other way.

Surviving College

by Jessica Duvall

I am 25 years old and live in Emporia, Kansas where I attend Emporia State University. I am getting my degree in Elementary Education/Early Childhood Education/Special Education. While attending school I currently work in the pharmaceutical field and substitute teach.

I was diagnosed with celiac disease on New Years Eve of 2002. I began my new life and lifestyle January 1, 2003. It is sort of ironic that the beginning of a new year was the beginning of a new life for me. It has been a great learning experience.

I am currently attending college so I'm going to offer a few tips on "surviving" the everyday stress of college and also dealing with celiac. A person with celiac CAN survive college. It just takes some extra effort and planning on your part.

The typical college diet usually consists of warm pizza, cold pizza, beer, sandwiches, doughnuts, and the occasional vegetable when you visit mom and dad. Instead of what I call "evil pizza from the Hut," I now make my own pizza using gluten-free pizza crusts and my favorite toppings. You can find crusts that are ready-made. Just top them and pop in the oven. They are not exactly the same but it sure does curb the cravings!

Beer and college go together but beer is a HUGE NO NO for celiacs. I believe they are working on a gluten-free version but it will be some time until it is out. In the meantime, have a glass of gluten-free champagne with your pizza. YUM!

Instead of a quick sandwich use gluten-free lunchmeat and make a roll up. Take the meat, put on cheese, mayo, lettuce, and other normal sandwich "fixin's" and roll it up. This is a great alternative to a sandwich and just as satisfying. Not to mention it is a quick meal and great for someone on the go.

Doughnuts are hard to replace. The doughnuts with gluten are so light and fluffy. I am afraid to tell you doughnuts are no longer light and fluffy. They can also double as paper weights for your homework, if necessary. However, they do not have a bad taste at all. They are a great substitute when you have that morning craving. Try them, you just might like them.

A student in college has little free time. If you do have free time, you like to relax and not have to worry about where your next meal is coming from. I personally have a few "tricks" so I get free time to sit down and relax. I try to do most of my cooking just one or two days a week. When I cook, I automatically make plenty of food so I have something to eat for more than just one day. I also take at least one portion out and put it into a plastic container for the freezer. I recommend getting some freezer tape and a marker. Use them to label all foods with the name and date cooked. You will thank yourself later when you can identify the frozen objects that all look alike when frozen.

I try to cook with recipes that fill all the food groups in one dish. Stir-frys are great. They even freeze very well and are good when reheated. Try to make entrees that have only a few ingredients, it just makes cooking easier and quicker.

All college students need cookies and sweets. I try to bake these as the cravings arise, but again make enough so that a portion or two can be frozen. Do not deny yourself something you crave. Find a gluten-free way to make it. Most recipes containing gluten ingredients can be adapted. Those evil elves are always on television trying to get us to have their cookies, but you can make cookies of your own that would knock the little socks off those elves. Take any "traditional" recipe. Substitute the flour with all purpose gluten-free flour, add some xanthum gum and follow the rest of the recipe. Pour yourself a glass of milk and enjoy!

If you are going to live in the dorms, make a point to meet with the people who are going to be providing your meals. You are covered under the Americans With Disabilities Act, and they MUST provide you with adequate foods. Sit down with the dietitian of the college and talk with him or her about your needs. They may also decide that giving you a room with your own kitchenette, or at least a room near one, is the best option. You might also decide living on your own is the best option for you and your needs. No matter what you decide, be sure to educate yourself about your needs and requirements. Enjoy your time in school!

My final thought: do not let celiac disease rule your life. Have fun but make your health a priority.

Coping With Celiac Disease In The Corporate World

by Laura Fairweather

I was diagnosed with celiac disease a few weeks before my 21st birthday. Now, six years into the diet, I've come a long way from the bummed out college senior who thought celiac stood for "Couldn't Eat Like I Always Could." A self-described carnivore in my pre gluten-free days, I now enjoy eating foods representing all food groups...as long as someone else cooks for me!

We all know the toughest part of keeping a gluten-free diet is eating away from home. My life would be much easier if I didn't have to work or I could work from home. But since I do spend five days a week in the "corporate world" (and a girl's got to eat!), I've learned to cope the best I can.

I work smack in the middle of Boston's financial district. We have two food courts, three taco/burrito joints, four fast food restaurants, Chinatown, two great Italian places and at least ten delis and they are all within a five minute walk of our office building. I've surveyed everywhere and maybe a handful of those places have one thing on their menu I can eat. Usually I'm a pretty good sport about being a celiac, but it never ceases to amaze me when my co-workers complain they're sick of eating the same thing for lunch everyday. That's when my little bitter side comes out! So you're hearing me whine (I'm assuming if you're reading this, you feel my pain) but I know only I have the power to make my situation better. The fact is I have celiac disease, and yes, the diagnosis comes with limitations. But how limited you actually are depends on how limited you are willing to be. Personally, I refuse to let celiac disease be a life-altering health condition. That said, I'd like to share some of my ideas:

Laura's Top 10 Gluten-Free Lunch Recommendations At The Office

1) **"Pasta Pizza"** – This is one of my favorite things to make for dinner at home. Next time you make gluten-free pasta for dinner, make double the amount you usually would. Eat the first half for dinner and then put the rest in a Tupperware dish (I find the long, flat, rectangular shaped ones work the best), cover it with your favorite pizza or marinara sauce and sprinkle shredded cheese on top. Bring it with you to work and after a minute in the microwave you have a great lunch. (Note: last time I did this everyone told me it looked and smelled great. They didn't know about my gluten-free diet.)

2) **Rice** – I always joke that I'm on the "Survivor Diet" because I eat so much rice. It may not seem like much of a meal but I find a large helping of steamed rice to be a great lunch, especially when you mix in some steamed vegetables. You can order it at any Chinese or Japanese restaurant or take-out stand. If you have a rice cooker at home (I strongly believe that every celiac should own a rice cooker), make a few cups of rice and bring some to work in your handy dandy Tupperware.

3) **Sandwiches** – Let's face it folks, these are no longer the days of "banana babies" when doctors and nutritionists thought the only thing celiac patients could eat were bananas. We're blessed to have quite a few vendors that make gluten-free breads and rolls. I have to say that in the six years I've been gluten-free I've seen a tremendous amount of new products, and they just keep getting better. There are several great gluten-free breads that you can order on the Internet. Sometimes I'll bring a loaf of bread to work at the beginning of the week and keep it in my company's kitchen freezer. At lunchtime, I just take out two slices, microwave them and make a sandwich, whether it's peanut butter and jelly (which is easy to keep at work), or gluten-free cold cuts. At first, it felt a little strange to assemble my

lunch at work, but I find that gluten-free bread is much better when eaten warm or freshly microwaved. As it turns out, in the past few months, I've caught plenty of my co-workers piecing their lunches together in our office kitchenette as well. My office freezer has loaves of wheat bread in addition to my gluten-free bread. I think whether you're gluten-free or not, it's simply easier to bring in all the ingredients at the beginning of the week and then you're all set.

4) **Stir-fry** (more leftovers) – Lucky for me my gem of a husband loves to cook dinner so I tend to have a lot of leftovers. But even before I was married and had a personal chef, I used to make stir-fry at home so I could bring it in for lunch the next day. Just mix meat/chicken/shrimp/tofu and your favorite vegetables or even just vegetables alone with a gluten-free sauce or marinade of your choice and you have a great meal. Add rice or rice noodles and you have an even bigger meal. Hint: a lot of Thai sauces (sold in your regular grocery store) are gluten-free.

5) **Smoothies** – These days everyone is on a health kick and I've seen a rise in the popularity of juice bars which used to be a West Coast thing. If there's somewhere near your office that specializes in smoothies, I

highly suggest you become a frequent customer. Peek around a bit and you'll notice that a lot of places include smoothies on their menus now (especially salad joints). Smoothies, which are typically a mix of fresh fruit, yogurt, and sorbet, can be quite a satisfying meal and they're also usually low fat. Avoid "boosters," or read ingredients carefully as these supplements often contain gluten. Also be careful of places that list smoothies on their menu but in reality just add flavored syrup to vanilla yogurt. They do not taste nearly as good and sometimes contain gluten.

6) **Fast Food/Wendy's** – In the first few years of my gluten-free diet I just couldn't do without McDonald's. I would go every other week or so and get a cheeseburger without a bun and french fries. Older age (I'm 26) and lack of exercise has forced me to mostly give up fast food, but I have to admit, I still frequent the Wendy's down the street from my office. Surprisingly Wendy's offers a number of gluten-free items on their menu and they're not all that bad for you. Try their chili, baked potato, or salads and every now and then treat yourself to a burger without a bun. Celiacs give up a lot of yummy food so we deserve an indulgence sometimes.

7) **Salad** – You can get salad pretty much anywhere these days. If you like to top your salad with tuna salad be careful because many delis add bread crumbs to their tuna. If there aren't any good places for salad in your work neighborhood, make your own at home and bring it in.

8) **Sushi** – Word on the street is sushi makes a terrific gluten-free meal (but watch out for fake crabmeat and bring your own soy sauce.). Personally I'm not a big sushi fan, but I wouldn't want to exclude it from this list.

9) **Pasta Salad** - Much like "Pasta Pizza" (see #1 above), making pasta salad can be very quick and easy if you think ahead when you make pasta for dinner. Boil gluten-free pasta (my pick: Tinkyada spirals), drain it, rinse for about 20 seconds with cold water while it's still in the strainer, then mix in your favorite gluten-free salad dressing. Add in some chopped up vegetables, cheese cubes, raisins, nuts, whatever you like, and you have yourself a delicious lunch for work. The greatest thing about pasta salad is you can make it in large amounts and it will last for days.

10) **Don't Be Shy**-Get to know your local food vendors. There's an Italian restaurant down the street from my office that people love

to go to for lunch. At first I shied away because nothing on their menu is gluten-free, but one day I was feeling brave (and hungry) and decided to talk to one of the chefs about my special needs. He was intrigued by my diet and made me a delicious chicken and vegetable dish in a gluten-free white wine sauce. Sure it took a few extra minutes, but it was well worth it, and I never would have received such a delicious meal if I didn't ask.

The last thought I'd like to leave you with is this: if I can handle a gluten-free diet anyone can. Trust me, I was absolutely crushed when I was diagnosed in college. I had avoided vegetables most of my life and was relying solely on frozen meals, fast food, and pizza. To this day I'm still amazed with myself. I eat a large variety of healthy foods. I handle my diet so well I have full faith that all of you can too. Just keep things in perspective and remember, if you have to have a disease, at least it's one so easily treated. Some people have much bigger things to worry about than not being able to eat at Dunkin' Donuts. ✒️

Out Of The Closet

by Christie Schroeter

Christie has also written "Knitting Your Body To Health," which can be read in Chapter Four.

Social circles revolve around food. They always have and probably always will. Never is it such a glaring fact as when you are diagnosed with celiac sprue. Suddenly you are confronted with explaining your dietary restrictions to old and new friends, relatives, and business associates. Just when you're trying to get the hang of gluten-free living, friends call to see if a movie and pizza would be a fun evening out. Then Aunt Margie asks you over for one of her home cooked meals, with hidden ingredients smothered into every morsel. There's always the potluck surprise at church. Who knows what mystery lurks in those mounds of food?

My way of coping at first was to become a "closet celiac." Don't admit there's a problem, avoid meal situations, and hope someone would suggest an activity that doesn't involve food. This never works. How long can you hide out? Invitations became less frequent and finally dwindled down to somewhere between rare and non-existent. After much soul searching I decided I wanted to fully participate in life and that meant coming to terms with the food issue. No more excuses. No more hiding.

When I'm asked out to lunch or dinner these days I explain I have dietary restrictions and then suggest a restaurant which I feel can work out an acceptable meal for me. That means calling ahead and talking to the chef or manager about the gluten-free items on the menu.

Potluck suppers are easy if I bring two large contributions to the meal I know I can eat. Very rarely do others notice I'm not partaking of the other selections. If they do, I quietly explain I'm on a strict diet, not elaborating anymore than I have to.

Showing up with tasty dishes at a family gathering also works well. Not only am I guaranteed food on my plate but it helps out the person who has no idea what to cook for me. I always strive to blend my contributions with whatever the hostess or host is serving. (Nothing like bringing chili when the entrée is filet mignon.)

It's a challenge living in a unique way in a gluten laden world. There's no doubt about it. But I discovered hiding behind my fears only served to separate me from enjoying the company of others. I find myself becoming more creative as time passes. This year I'm planning to invite friends for some short day trips in the car to scenic areas. Doesn't a picnic lunch sound like fun?

Don't Keep Celiac Disease A Secret

by Leslie Elsner

After three years of wasting away and a friendly pat on the shoulder from a GI who thought I needed a shrink (Quack!), I received my celiac disease diagnosis in October 1994. I spent 10 years as an active member of the Westchester Celiac Support Group where I wrote the "hand holding" sections of the newsletter, as well as serving on the board. I see celiac disease as a challenge that can only be met with a smile, a positive attitude, and ongoing sense of humor.

I s it just me or are others finding celiacs in the oddest places? I just had to share my story of how, in the last four days, I came across three new celiacs. Ironically, all through my well-informed non-celiac friend, Laura.

Encounter 1: One of Laura's friends calls to say 'hi' and mentions he has been very ill and has just finally received a diagnosis but is still feeling sick in his gut. Laura mentions maybe he should ask his doctor to test him for celiac disease. There is dead silence on the other end of the phone and then her friend says, "That's what I have and what do you know about celiac disease?"

Encounter 2: I join Laura down at her shore house this weekend. As I am showering she quietly asks one of the housemates who is in charge of the BBQ if he wouldn't mind cleaning off a portion of the grill. She explains her friend has severe food allergies and can't eat off the spot where barbecue sauce had just been. He looks at her with a strange look and asks, "What kind of allergies?" Laura answers, "She's a celiac and can't have something called gluten." He looks amazed and says, "Laura, that's funny, I'm a celiac too. I was diagnosed eight years ago."

Encounter 3: I arrive at the table and get into a full discussion of celiac disease with my new celiac buddy. A visitor to the house sits down and says, "Excuse me for intruding, but I have a question. My sister-in-law doesn't have celiac disease but she has something called severe gluten intolerance and they sometimes call it sprue. Would you mind if I ask you some questions for her?" Is that weird or what?

The moral of the story: Don't keep celiac disease a secret. Spread the word, inform those around you, and tell them about the celiac e-mail list and the support groups and vendors that are available to us. I can't tell you the relief I saw on those faces when they realized they are not alone. I think it's coming closer to a time where celiac disease may be the "in disease" (not that I wish it on anyone). But gosh, many people can be saved from a great deal of suffering and isolation! ✍️

Should I Or Shouldn't I?

by Christine Gill

I am a 37-year-old devoted mother to a wonderful, smart, loving son named Corey. I love him very much.

I am also an artist who loves to create unique and special floral pieces. I feel healthy again by sticking to my special diet; my special gluten-free diet.

This story is dedicated to my brother, Michael, whom I admire. I relate to his struggles every day and I love him very much

Should I eat that wonderful piece of vanilla cake offered to me at a party or shouldn't I? I ask this question over and over to myself each day through my years of dealing with celiac disease. It seems I am always in this type of dilemma or situation and it's very frustrating. I want to say "yes," but I know how I would feel if I do. In a matter of only a few hours I will feel horrible. A nauseous feeling will take over, cramps will arrive, and that wonderful feeling of being car sick, as I call it, will have the best of me. Sometimes it will take days to feel better again or normal. Do I really want to feel like this? Is having this piece of delicious cake worth it to me? No, to me it's not. So, I refuse, again and again.

My name is Christine. I am 37 years of age and this is my story. Three years ago I suffered with dermatitis hepetiformis. I asked myself why my skin was doing this, I never had these horrible itchy rashes before. Where are they coming from now? For months I suffered. At my first visit with a dermatologist, he told me it was dermatitis hepetiformis and all I needed to do was apply the creams he would prescribe. What he didn't tell me was that in my case it was caused by gluten.

So for months I applied the prescribed creams to the "rash patches" or "raised bumps with clear liquid in them" as I always called them. It didn't give much relief. The itching was so bad at times, I couldn't deal with it. It was worse than poison ivy. When I scratched the areas, it felt like raised skin and not normal. It also felt warm to the touch. It was all over my body, on both my knees, on the side of my legs, elbows, arms, buttocks, in my scalp, and then on my face. I think that was the last straw, when my skin broke out on my face. I was so embarrassed to go anywhere.

I tried hiding the patches on my face with makeup. Then when I did go out, I prayed I didn't see anyone I knew. This continued for months. I felt alienated and depressed and ugly! The medicated creams were not doing the job. I knew something was just not right.

Then things in my life started getting a bit more complicated. Through my years I was always thin and petite. Being five feet eight inches tall I looked very skinny. I never had a problem with whatever I ate. All my friends wanted to know what my secret for staying so thin was. I ate well, exercised, and stayed active, but I couldn't gain weight for anything. Over the years it seemed I always had an irregular bowel movement, but I never really paid too much attention to it. It seemed kind of abnormal going maybe three to four times a day, but that's how it was for years. To me I thought it was normal. Then I had days when I was stressed out or was very nervous about something. On those days I went more often. On top of my health problems I was dealing with my son Corey's type 1 diabetes diagnosis, as well as watching my older brother struggle with Crohn's disease.

I had no idea what celiac disease was. He said, "Try not to eat any wheat flour." I was so unprepared for this. "Are you kidding me? Do you mean bread?" ... He explained to me about the foods I couldn't eat. I was shocked.

I was emotionally and mentally finished. I had asked God, "Why is this happening?" I dedicated all of my time to Corey and his health. I had to deal with hospitals, doctors, insulin, needles, blood sugar monitors, and unanswered questions. My health situation, or whatever I was experiencing was put on hold. I was so angry and frustrated with the world. Every time someone asked me about Corey I would cry. I just couldn't talk about it. I still cry today. I think about the other children in the world that have cancer, leukemia, etc. and say, "Well at least Corey doesn't have that." But still it's a struggle. I pray that someone will come up with a cure.

As time went on I started to get really sick. It was so bad I couldn't even leave the house. Diarrhea, bloating, cramps, etc. and all the lovely things that go with celiac disease took over my body. Every morning I would eat my favorite, Farina, but it went right through me, literally! Whatever I ate seemed not to stay in, so to speak. I started to lose weight, badly. I was very skinny, skinnier than ever. My clothes wouldn't fit. I truly looked anorexic. I felt like giving up. Between Corey's situation and my so-called sickness, I felt alone. "Why is this happening?"

Well, I finally made an appointment with a gastroenterologist. I couldn't even sit comfortably in his office while I waited until it was my turn. I had to find the bathroom, of course. After my examination, an appointment was made for a colonoscopy for a couple of days away.

Ideas poured into my head. Do I have what my brother is struggling with all these years? I knew what my brother was going through. Suffering and not having control of his body was his everyday life. I cried again. I think the preparation and the actual procedure was the worst thing I experienced. For some, they say, "really?...it wasn't that bad." But for me it was horrible. I think because I was so skinny, the doctor just couldn't turn his scope the way he wanted.

I went on the Internet again. I couldn't believe there were sites on celiac disease. Other people were going through the same thing I was. I could read the frustrations in their e-mails, like how I was feeling.

It hurt even though I was "under." The good thing was my intestines looked good. He said I had irritable bowel syndrome, not Crohn's. I was so relieved. I was so happy. He also said I have to be on a specific diet and there's a lot of information on the Internet, so I could read up on it. He prescribed some medication so I would feel better. I also was supposed to return to his office for a follow-up a few days later. When I returned for the follow-up he looked at my chart and my blood results. He said, "Well I know I told you have irritable bowel syndrome, but it seems you tested very high on the celiac test."

I had no idea what celiac disease was. He said, "Try not to eat any wheat flour." I was so unprepared for this. "Are you kidding me? Do you mean bread?" He said, "Well there's more to it than just bread." He explained to me about the foods I couldn't eat. I was shocked. I was also frustrated his first diagnosis was incorrect.

Then I thought about it. I mean I love all kinds of breads. What I didn't realize was I would also have to give up pretzels, which is one my favorite foods, but that was just the beginning. Then the list went on and on with what I couldn't eat. I was like, "I can't do this." Now I was really angry. I cried again leaving the doctor's office as I thought about all the things made of wheat flour. While driving home, I was speechless.

After months went by, I tried my hardest not to eat anything with wheat flour in it. I think I made my local health food store very rich. I wondered if I should buy some stock, then we could both be rich. I was blessed because I had learned the manager of my local health store was also celiac. I thought, "you're kidding?" She told me what types of products were gluten-free and which brands were good. She helped me out a lot. I asked questions, lots of them. I went on the Internet again. I couldn't believe there were sites on celiac disease. Other people were going through the same thing I was. I could read the frustrations in their e-mails, like how I was feeling. I couldn't believe it.

I tried to read as much information as I could about celiac disease. It's funny because as I started the gluten-free diet my skin started to clear up. I was amazed. I also started to feel better. I mean the diarrhea was still there, but not as bad. I went from going to the little girl's room from maybe ten times a day to two or three times. Some days, depending on what I was dealing with, I only went once. I actually could leave the house again and not have to worry about where a bathroom was located. It was such a relief!

So, to end my story, there is relief out there if you are strong, like me. Stay positive and don't give up. Keep asking questions. Visit your local health food store and ask for their gluten-free foods. There may also be support groups in your local area. The Internet can also be a big help. You can feel better if you stick to your guns and to your special diet. If you travel, bring your gluten-free foods with you. It's easier and more convenient.

Sorry, but you just can't eat the piece of cake waiting for you at that party. However, bring your own gluten-free cake. That's all. You'll feel better, literally! ✍

CHAPTER

10

Travel
Tales

*Don't Forget To Pack
Your Gluten-Free Food*

> *Vacations are something I crave,*
> *If prepared I don't have to be brave.*
> *Pack the gluten-free meal,*
> *It's not a big deal.*
> *To my diet I won't be a slave.*

Traveling With Celiac Disease
by Michael Neiberg

I am a Professor of History at the United States Air Force Academy in Colorado Springs. After a long battle with a variety of symptoms, I was diagnosed with celiac disease in April 2002 at age 33. I live in Colorado Springs with my wife and two daughters and I travel wherever and whenever I can.

E very person with celiac disease must have a moment like the one I had in Lyon, France, in 2001. I did not yet know I had celiac disease but I knew something was wrong. At this point I had been incorrectly diagnosed with complex migraines and told to avoid red wine, hard cheese, coffee, and second-hand cigarette smoke. I traveled to France despite these seemingly awesome restrictions. I was loaded with migraine medicines and determined to avoid the forbidden items as much as possible. Of course, bread was not on the forbidden list and I remember my first two meals in France were a bag of pastries and a baguette sandwich.

Needless to say after a few days of this diet I began to feel sicker and sicker. I managed to give the presentation, which was the reason for my going to France but could barely leave my hotel room for two days afterward. I missed the conference dinner and most of the later sessions. I knew I was prone to anxiety attacks as a side effect of exposure to gluten. Lying in a mediocre French hotel I was sick and terrified for my life which only increased these anxieties.

My basic approach to this trip involved bringing gluten-free meal replacement bars for breakfast, eating an early lunch, keeping fruit and candy with me for snacks, and then eating a big dinner.

I called the airline to inquire about changing my ticket for the next available flight, meaning I would miss the chance to visit with friends in Paris. My wife, who was in Colorado, talked me out of leaving early and I finished the trip. I was determined never to travel again, no matter how much I enjoyed it, or how important it was to my career.

The doctors did not diagnose me with celiac disease until the following April. Shortly after the diagnosis I was asked to go back to France for ten days. I accepted but had mixed feelings. On the one hand, I was apprehensive given my last experience. On the other, I had a renewed determination to travel with this disease and to live my life my way. I was traveling with a group that had never been to France and I was responsible for their safety and for making sure we accomplished what we had been sent to do. Still unsure about everything I needed to avoid, I assembled the group at my house before leaving and explained the disease. I asked them to help me avoid anything that might contain wheat, barley, oats, or rye. They graciously agreed and were a tremendous help to me.

My basic approach to this trip involved bringing gluten-free meal replacement bars for breakfast, eating an early lunch, keeping fruit and candy with me for snacks, and then eating a big dinner. At restaurants, I asked to speak to the owner or head chef and explained what I needed. Most French restaurants were quite accommodating. The owner of one of them (Le Rapier, on the smaller town square in Arras) told me in France an allergy or disease should never prevent someone from getting a good meal. Although France does not understand celiac disease as well as many other countries, that philosophy helped a lot. I was still very worried about cross-contamination or eating

> *In my view, celiac disease should not prevent anyone from enjoying travel, although there will be difficult moments and the risk of accidental exposure is always present.*

something that contained an unnoticed source of gluten, but I had no problems on this trip and I enjoyed myself tremendously.

Since then I have made three more overseas trips that have taken me to England, France and Sweden. In general, the British and the Scandinavians understand celiac disease extremely well. I never had a problem in either place. Several British menus even indicated which foods were gluten-free. I avoided pubs, except those that served the ubiquitous "jacket potato," a gluten-free lifeline for a quick, cheap meal. The disease is not well known in France and if you do not speak French I recommend printing a card that will read something like:

"J'ai la maladie coeliac, une maladie rare, mais sérieux. Il me faut strictement eviter tous produits provenant du blé, orge, avoin, et seigle. Veuillez m'indiquer quels plats ne contient pas les ingrédients interdit pour mon régime. Merci de votre comprehension."

(Translation: I have celiac disease, a rare but serious condition. I must carefully avoid all products made from wheat, barley, oats, and rye. Would you please indicate to me the products on your menu that are safe for my diet. Thank you for your understanding.)

A translation card is generally not necessary in Scandinavia, where English is widely understood.

Recently, my wife, daughter and I spent one month in West Sussex, England, and one month in Paris. I used to have problems watching friends and family eat pastries or bread in front of me, but no more. I have learned to enjoy what I can.

In June 2003, I went to a conference at Oxford sponsored by the same group that had met in Lyon in 2001. By the time of the 2003 meeting, I had gained back almost thirty pounds and was in much better physical shape. As in 2001, I gave my presentation. Unlike 2001, however, I was healthy and therefore able to participate fully in all of the conference's activities. The conference dinner was held at a Lebanese restaurant that fully understood celiac disease. The owner brought out the dishes family style, carefully pointing out to me what I could eat and what I needed to avoid. On the way out of the restaurant, I approached him and thanked him for his hospitality and his concern for my diet. He replied, "No need to thank me. It is my job." On the way back to my hotel I reflected on the differences between my health at the two conferences and the remarkable progress I had made.

In my view, celiac disease should not prevent anyone from enjoying travel, although there will be difficult moments, and the risk of accidental exposure is always present. Here are my suggestions about traveling with celiac disease. I hope they help.

1) Check Web sites before you leave. Almost all European countries have a celiac Web site that can give you information about where to buy food. Many will list celiac-friendly restaurants and list the foods to be avoided in the local language. The Italian version lists restaurants owned by celiac chefs.

2) Bring food with you. An assortment of meal replacement bars will be invaluable. There are also several gluten-free instant meals that are well worth bringing with you.

3) Check with your airline to see if it offers gluten-free meals. In general, European carriers are more likely to offer a gluten-free meal, although many American carriers still do. British Airways and SAS were both very accommodating. One American carrier

served a "gluten-free" meal of pasta of unknown origin, and multi-grain crackers that were most definitely NOT gluten-free. Be safe and put some gluten-free food in your carry-on bag.

4) When eating in restaurants ask careful, probing questions. If the server seems confused, ask to speak to the chef. In Oxford, England, a chef actually came out of the kitchen with a crayon and lined out the foods on the menu which contained gluten. Of course, it is best to go when the restaurant is not busy. Stop by the restaurant during its quiet hours to make a reservation for later and determine if the staff understands your needs.

5) Find grocery stores near you. Major chains like Waitrose and Tesco in Britain, and Monoprix in France carry gluten-free items. Marks and Spencer in Britain label gluten and wheat as allergens on their packaging. There are also natural food stores like Naturalia and La Vie Claire, and even some pharmacies that carry gluten-free food. Pharmacies are an outstanding source of information on gluten-free resources, even providing lists of terms. Moreover, most pharmacies in Europe have at least one person who speaks English.

6) If you plan to stay in a city for longer than a few days, look to rent a place with a kitchen. Many hotels offer kitchenettes and in most cities you can rent an apartment for short or long term. You will save money by not eating out as often and you will be able to control what you eat. You will also have the pleasure of shopping at the local markets, which can be a real treat.

If you are still nervous about going overseas due to celiac disease, I recommend you start with a trip to Great Britain or Sweden. I saw butcher shops that had their sausages labeled gluten-free, grocery stores with dedicated gluten-free aisles, and I had wonderful gluten-free meals served to me in both places. I only encountered clueless kitchen staffs in British pubs. In restaurants, I never had the least difficulty. In fact, I have had a much easier time traveling in these two countries than I have traveling in the United States. I will continue to travel and have a trip to China planned in a few months. Celiac disease can take away some of my favorite foods but I am determined that it will not take away my ability to travel. As always, it is up to you to determine the level of exposure you want to risk but I say, "Bon Voyage."

A Disney World Vacation
by Joyce Etheridge

My son and I were diagnosed with celiac in March 2000. It was a major challenge for us to change our way of eating. When we got the gluten out of us we discovered we were allergic to corn and dairy as well. If that wasn't enough I was also diagnosed with candida and had to give up yeast, sugar, citric acid, canola oil, carbs, beef, and fruit. It was very hard for me to give everything up at once. With a good friend's help, both my son and I have learned the diet. Today we are doing really well.

After being diagnosed with celiac disease my family and I decided to visit Disney World for our vacation. It was our first trip to the Magic Kingdom and we were totally impressed with everything and decided to try to go back every year.

Knowing that I had to eat a certain way, I called in advance to make meal reservations and was surprised that gluten intolerance was in the computer system as a common food allergy. Now they have added celiac. I was advised to contact the chefs of each restaurant a few days prior to eating there so they would have time to order whatever food they didn't ordinarily carry. The more time you give them the better. I suggest you do this from home so when you're at the resort you can concentrate on the attractions you want to visit and not worry about what you're going to eat. It's a good plan but you know the old saying about "the best laid plans." This past year I could not get through to the Crystal Palace before we left on our trip. I also tried when we got down to Disney World but still wasn't able to get through on the telephone. I ended up going to the restaurant without contacting the chef but I'm happy to say that he was able to accommodate us.

When we arrived at Disney World we were very impressed with the food. We were also impressed to find that when we arrived at a restaurant the chef came to our table to meet and discuss everything with us. This is good because it gives you a chance to double check everything with the chef to avoid any problems. We then placed our orders and they were either made up special for us or, as sometimes was the case, the food was already cooking in the kitchen. They know to prepare our food independently from the other meals to avoid cross-contamination. At some places the chef would bring our food to us himself and at the end of the meal he would come back and make sure everything was okay. When you go to a table service restaurant, you'll want to allow at least an hour for meals as it takes time to be seated, have the chef come out to greet you, fix your food, and eat. It can be a long wait, but it's worth it in the end.

We have also discovered the character meals in the table service restaurants can accommodate the gluten-free diet. Just give the restaurant a few days notice. Also, if you plan to revisit a particular restaurant during your stay at Disney World, I would suggest you discuss any future meals with the chef at your first visit. The chefs will plan ahead for you and order any food you may want. Again, just to be safe, double check everything with the chef. Several times we have gone into restaurants and the chef on duty didn't know we were coming because the head chef did not pass our menu on to him. This is a very good reason to double check everything. It doesn't take long and it's worth it.

Even though Disney World is very well versed on celiac disease, you still need to be responsible for yourself and take nothing for granted. At one restaurant the cook was going to use rice dream milk in the mashed potatoes for my son. I told him there is .002% gluten in the milk. It is stated on the carton. It doesn't seem like much but we know it doesn't take much. Just ask them to bring the container out to you so you can read the labels for yourself. They are very willing to do this and you have the right to question ingredients the chef will use to prepare your food. Another time, my son ate pancakes made with corn flour and got sick. I should have checked the ingredients myself on the pancakes for corn in them.

We've gone back to Disney World for the past three years and our family has favorite restaurants to recommend. A few suggestions are Chef Mickey in the Contemporary Hotel, Crystal Palace at Magic Kingdom, Liberty Tree Tavern at Magic Kingdom, Sci-Fi Dine-in Theater at MGM Studios, 50's Prime Time Cafe at MGM Studios and Restaurantosaurus at Animal Park. This is a character breakfast in the morning and turns into McDonald's for lunch and dinner. Throughout the parks the hot dogs are gluten-free along with corn free. They also have McDonald's french fry stands throughout some parks where all they serve are fries and drinks so there is no cross-contamination with other fried foods. We have a dairy allergy along with corn allergy, so I don't know whether the ice cream in the parks is gluten-free or not.

We found the resorts of Disney World extremely accommodating to us, not only when it came to food, but also to our room. Because of my allergies I've learned to be concerned about soaps and cleaning supplies used in hotels, so I discussed this with the head of Housekeeping. I told her I was worried about some of the chemicals. She was very nice and researched the brands of the resort's laundry soap and other cleaning supplies commonly used. Rather than worry about the products, we agreed it would be best to wash our towels in pure hot water and clean our room without using chemicals. Honestly, I don't know how they did it, but everything was clean and we never had a bad reaction. Now whenever I make our travel reservations I'm certain to ask that no chemicals be used to clean the room and our towels be washed in soap-free hot water.

One last thing to be aware of is how and where to get medical attention on Disney property, just in case you need it. There are doctors on Disney property and they can make house calls if you wish.

These are just some of my family's experiences at Disney World and I wanted to share them so other people who want to experience Disney World can do so and not worry about being able to eat. We have had a few setbacks but in the end our family says Disney World is the number one vacation place to go for a gluten-free diet. We have gone three years in a row and are looking forward to another trip.

Doing Disney World Gluten-Free

by Donna Griffin

By day, I am a special education teacher in a large public middle school. By day and night, I am a mom of three "children," 27, 21, and 16. By coincidence, several months after our oldest daughter's (Jennifer) diagnosis, as a result of our family screening and my consequent biopsy, I too was diagnosed with celiac disease! By luck, Jen and I both had the good fortune of becoming part of a strong support network through the Westchester Celiac Sprue Support Group.

When we first made vacation plans to go to Disney World, our biggest dilemma was whether to drive to Orlando and save ourselves some money or to fly and splurge a little. However, several months later, our just "sweet" sixteen-year-old daughter, Jennifer, was diagnosed with celiac disease. Suddenly, the dilemma became whether to go at all!

As parents of a newly diagnosed celiac we had our own issues to deal with and after many months of Jennifer being ill, we were all emotionally drained. As her mom, I was determined to show Jennifer (and frankly myself as well) her life would be "normal," even without gluten. So began Jennifer's first sojourn as a celiac.

Our first step was to call the Celiacs of Orlando Support Group. They were very helpful and suggested I contact the executive chefs at each of the theme parks. I was still naive enough to think someone at the central reservations number at Disney would surely have these phone numbers available. After several phone calls, I finally became aware of a special requests reservation person. Her name was Linda and she magically (no pun intended) began to make things happen. She arranged for a refrigerator to be in the room at no extra charge, provided a brand new, still in the box, unopened toaster, and assisted me in making special gluten-free and lactose-free meal reservations sixty days in advance at full service Disney restaurants. Perhaps most importantly, Linda provided me with the names and numbers of the (mysterious) executive chefs. She also e-mailed the concierge at the Disney resort where we were staying and advised them they needed to get some gluten-free and lactose-free items in stock. However, this was not in place when we arrived so I made an unhappy Mouseketeer phone call. Shortly thereafter someone from guest relations at the resort went to Chamberlain's and brought gluten-free waffles, cookies, and Lactaid milk directly to our room.

So now everything seemed to be in place. Well, you know what they say about the best laid plans... As luck would have it, there was a lightning storm in central Florida the day we arrived, resulting in no natural gas for two days. This became an excuse at several locations and a really good way to get me fired up, with or without the gas! I made an early morning call to Brenda, the executive chef at the Magic Kingdom, who seemed genuinely upset at Jennifer's circumstance. Thankfully the gas crisis was also over at this point. She e-mailed all of the remaining restaurants, even if they were in Epcot or MGM, putting them on a sort of "alert." Ultimately, this led to chefs personally contacting either Jennifer or myself and pre-ordering her meal.

Even after this, there were still some rough spots but good help was available. Marianne, the executive chef at MGM, was very helpful after Brenda contacted her. She had done some work with the celiac support group in Orlando, and knew enough to try to coordinate Jennifer's meals at MGM so there was some variety. Chef Wendy at the Prime Time Cafe was especially thoughtful in her service. Although there is an executive chef at Epcot, the communication was weak and we had a less than pleasant experience arranging for a much awaited gluten-free and lactose-free Mexican meal. Ironically, the restaurant that was the most accommodating had the least amount of notice and was the only place Jennifer chose to go to more than once: Spoodles on the Disney Boardwalk. The chef was Damian and he really went out of his way to make a special dinner and a gluten-free and lactose-free fruit cobbler for dessert.

Magic Kingdom restaurants also deserve some accolades. Cinderella's Royal Table served Jennifer a gluten-free and lactose-free breakfast fit for a queen. Someone at Tony's Town Square hightailed it over to Adventureland to get a Dole Whip for dessert (there are two types; the one with no ice cream is gluten-free and lactose-free....yes, I called Dole beforehand).

Before I leave the Magic Kingdom, some gluten-free trivia: The french fries at Casey's at the end of Main Street are gluten-free, as is the Magic Kingdom popcorn; and there is gluten-free ice cream at the Cone Shop on Main Street. Several of the full service restaurants had Tofutti on hand for us.

My best advice would be always to speak directly to the chef, have some emergency rations on hand just in case, and consider a condo or room with a kitchenette. 🖎

Donna's daughter, Jennifer, has written "When You're A Teen," which can be read in Chapter Seven.

Steps For Planning A Vacation
by Jessica Duvall

Jessica has written "Surviving College," which can be read in Chapter Nine, a recipe for "Lemon Curd," which can be found in Chapter 11, and "Keep A Food Diary," which can be read in Chapter 12.

Planning a vacation can be stressful, especially for someone with celiac disease. Here are a few tips I've found to be helpful:

* Bake cookies ahead of time. Freeze them and place them in individual bags.

* Buy paper plates, bowls, and silverware to bring along.

* Take along a George Foreman grill.

* Book a hotel room with a small kitchenette and microwave. Use the microwave in the hotel to warm up Thai noodles, soup, or whatever else.

* Find a good grocery store when you arrive at your destination. Purchase fresh veggies, fruits, and meat to cook on your George Foreman grill.

* Locate a health food store that sells goodies, in case you forgot something.

* Purchase gluten-free goodies ahead of time so you don't have the expense of purchasing them all at once.

* Take prepared gluten-free pantry pizza crust and hopefully a pizza place will put toppings on for you without too much argument. However, be careful of cross-contamination

* Take a cooler that you can pack with lunch meats and cheeses. Bring along gluten-free crackers for easy lunches.

* Call ahead and locate restaurants that aren't scared of having a person with celiac disease in their place of business.

* Take soy crisps, peanut butter, and boxes of cereal you like for breakfast.

If you prepare properly you can enjoy your vacation and not focus on foods.

Recipes
For
Success

Now You're Cooking

[
You don't need to feel so deprived,
It isn't that hard to survive.
The recipes here,
Will bring you good cheer.
With so many foods you will thrive.
]

My Horrific
Baking Experience
by Cristina Bourgard

I'm in my early twenties and currently working on a Master's Degree in Social Work. Between studying, working, planning a wedding, and dealing with celiac, I'm a very busy person! I've had lots of support from my family and friends who are now all proficient in finding gluten-free products. To all of my family and friends, I would like to say, "THANK YOU"!

I was diagnosed with celiac disease recently, so I am still a novice when it comes to gluten-free baking. My first attempt at a loaf of buckwheat raisin bread turned out to be like a horrific experiment from a B-rated science fiction movie. The loaf ended up being sticky with a pinkish-gray tinge. It weighed about a thousand pounds and tasted like dirt.

I bribed my family members to try this monstrosity (they tasted it to be good sports). Most of them ended up choking on the raisin-dirt flavor. My mom shouted, "eeeewwwwaaahhh" and heaved the bread into the garbage.

My second gluten-free baking attempt was to be sweet

rice bread. The mixture was gelatinous and gooey and refused to bake. After 40 minutes in the oven, I had created the sweet rice bread that took over Tokyo. It was more like "The Blob" than any loaf of bread I had ever seen. It was so rubbery it bounced on the floor (it also smelled musty).

My mother took pity on me and managed to create a gluten-free version of her wonderful banana bread. My family liked it (including my fussy father and boyfriend, who deem themselves "food experts"). I hope it helps you to not have to go though what I did to bake gluten-free.

Christina's Mom's Awesome
Gluten-Free Banana Bread

Ingredients:
  1 cup soy flour
  ¼ cup milk
  ½ cup potato starch flour
  ½ cup oil
  ¼ cup rice flour
  2 jumbo eggs
  ¼ cup garfava flour
  2 very ripe mashed bananas
  ½ teaspoon xanthum gum
  1½ cups sugar
  1 teaspoon baking soda
  1¼ teaspoons cream of tartar
  dash of salt
  ½ teaspoon each of cloves, cinnamon, nutmeg, allspice

Directions:

*Combine all dry ingredients, except sugar, into a large bowl.

*Combine eggs, milk, sugar, and bananas into another mixing bowl and beat until vaguely smooth (the bananas will still remain a bit lumpy).

*Turn the mixer on low and slowly add the dry ingredients. Beat until mixed (about 2 - 3 minutes).

*Pour into a 9 x 5 inch loaf pan and bake at 350 degrees for approximately one hour.

Hamburg Pie

by Tina Ackerman

Tina has also written "Long Road To Diagnosis," which can be read in Chapter One.

This recipe is a dish my mom made when I was a child. I have slightly adapted it to make it a quick, easy, gluten-free dinner. Leftovers reheat very well, which is a necessity for someone with celiac.

Hamburg Pie
(serves 4 - 6)

Ingredients:

- 1½ pounds ground beef
- 1 large egg
- ¼ cup gluten-free bread crumbs
- 1 12 ounce can gluten-free tomato sauce
- instant rice
- 1 cup shredded mozzarella cheese
- dash of pepper

Directions:

    *Preheat oven to 350 degrees.

    *In a medium bowl mix the ground beef, beaten egg, dash of pepper, and gluten-free bread crumbs.

    *Press the ground beef mixture into a 9 inch deep dish pie pan to make a "crust."

    *Pour the can of tomato sauce into the crust.

    *Rinse the tomato can and fill it with instant rice.

    *Pour the rice into the crust.

    *Fill the tomato can three-quarters full with water and pour the water into the crust.

    *Without disturbing the ground beef crust gently mix in the tomato rice mixture.

    *Tightly cover the pie pan with foil and place into the oven for 40 minutes.

    *Remove the pie from the oven and uncover.

    *Sprinkle cheese over the top of the pie, and without covering, place back into the oven until the cheese melts.

    *Let cool 5 minutes before cutting into slices.

    *Serve with a side of vegetables.

    *Recipe can also be doubled and cooked in a 9x14 inch casserole dish.

Pizalle Recipe
by Susan Hodges

Susan has also written "Baby Turkey," which can be read in Chapter Six and has contributed the recipe for Italian Sausage Rice Stuffing, which can also be found in this chapter.

In the years since our daughter, Hannah Rose, was diagnosed, we have tried to make things as normal (whatever that is) as possible. One of my fondest memories is of my mom baking oodles of pizalles. It's a traditional Italian Christmas cookie, baked in an iron similar to a waffle iron. I was always fascinated by the way it was sooo thin yet had a spider web design on one side and a floral design on the other...as a kid it was...magic! I did some research and found a pizalle maker for only $39.99 (I paid $80 for mine a couple of years ago) available in the Chef's catalog (chefscatalog.com or 1-800-338-3232). Here is the recipe we developed for the best tasting gluten-free or any other pizalle recipe!

(Please use a dedicated gluten-free pizalle iron to avoid cross-contamination)

Pizalle
(Makes about 40 cookies)

Ingredients:

> 6 extra large eggs (or 7 large eggs) at room temperature
> 3 - 3½ cups gluten-free Pantry French Bread/Bagel Mix (I am not affiliated with them in any way but they have made my life easier)
> 1 cup (½ pound) butter, melted, cooled to room temperature
> 1½ cups sugar
> 3 - 4 teaspoons gluten-free baking powder
> 2 tablespoons gluten-free vanilla

Directions:

> *In a large mixing bowl, use mixer to beat eggs until smooth.
> *Add sugar and beat until blended (1 minute).
> *Add cooled butter, gluten-free baking powder, and vanilla. Blend until smooth.
> *Stir in gluten-free flour mixture slowly, spoonful by spoonful until well blended.
> *Meanwhile heat your pizalle iron, spray with gluten-free non-stick spray.
> *Add 1 heaping tablespoon of mixture to each side of iron.
> *Close and lock iron. Release when steaming decreases (about 1 minute).
> *Lift off with fork to a cooling sheet.
> *Trim as cooled and stack.

Italian Sausage Rice Stuffing

by Susan Hodges

Susan has also written "Baby Turkey," which can be read in Chapter Six and has contributed another recipe for Pizalle, which can also be found in this chapter.

Italian Sausage
Rice Stuffing

Ingredients:

3 cups brown rice

½ - 1 cup wild rice

2 - 4 mild Italian sausages in casings

5½ cups water

2 tablespoons butter

1 tablespoon oil

2 - 3 tablespoons chicken soup mix (I use the Nutrimax brand)

1 - 2 stalks of celery finely chopped

1 medium onion finely chopped

2 - 3 cloves of garlic finely chopped (or to taste-we love garlic!)

1 bunch of parsley chopped

salt and pepper to taste

Directions:

*Add rice, water, 1 tablespoon butter, soup base, and some parsley to your rice cooker or sauce pan. We usually cook for about 45 minutes. Set aside.

*Melt 1 tablespoon butter and 1 tablespoon oil in skillet.

*When melted, add garlic and swirl it in the butter and oil mix. Add onion and sauté on medium-low until soft.

*Add celery. Sauté until soft.

*Add some parsley and swirl around until it is limp (not long).

*Add salt and pepper as desired.

*Set aside in another container.

*Using the same skillet, remove the sausage casings and brown the sausage so it doesn't get too crispy. Break into small, crumbled pieces as it cooks. Set aside.

*In a large mixing bowl combine all ingredients. Mix well, adjust seasoning to taste, cover and let the seasonings meld for 15 - 30 minutes.

*Stuff your bird of choice or bake at 350 degrees for about 30 minutes or until it looks ready.

Enjoy

Apple Pie
by Pam Gordon

My name is Pam and my husband Ben has celiac disease. He was diagnosed about five years ago after two years of testing. His doctor finally did the small intestine biopsy because he was running out of things for which to test! Ben handles his diet restrictions pretty well most of the time, but he misses sweets the most which is why I'm always coming up with dessert recipes.

Here is a recipe I like. It is an old recipe and all that had to be changed was the type of flour used for the crust. I brought this to a covered dish supper and was asked for the recipe.

Apple Pie

Ingredients:
Filling:
4 - 5 apples (peeled and sliced)
3 tablespoons water
2/3 cup cinnamon/sugar mixture
Topping:
1 cup gluten-free flour
½ cup brown sugar
½ cup butter

Directions:
> *Grease a large, glass pie pan.
> *Add apples and sprinkle water over them.
> *Sprinkle with cinnamon/sugar mixture.
> *Mix topping ingredients and crumble over top.
> *Bake at 350 degrees for 30 to 40 minutes.
> *Serve warm.

Cinnamon Crisps
by Kathleen Johe

Kathleen has also written "Anything For Our Children," which can be found in Chapter Six.

I created this cookie from a non gluten-free recipe I have used for years. My husband and son are crazy about cinnamon, so it was a necessary invention. It can be modified to chocolate by replacing the cinnamon with cocoa powder and the cinnamon chips with chocolate. Use fine ground Asian style rice flour for best results. Those who have issues with potato flour can substitute with rice flour, but add ¼ teaspoon more xanthan gum. Also, for those with dairy issues, you can use butter flavor Crisco instead of real butter.

Cinnamon Crisps
(Makes 2 dozen cookies)

Ingredients:
- 4 ounces butter, cold
- 1 cup sugar
- 1 teaspoon gluten-free vanilla extract
- 2 teaspoons cinnamon
- 1 egg

½ cup rice flour
¼ cup tapioca flour
¼ cup potato starch flour
1 teaspoon xanthan gum
½ teaspoon gluten-free baking powder
½ teaspoon gluten-free baking soda
¾ cup cinnamon baking chips, optional

Directions:

*Beat butter and ¾ cup sugar until light and fluffy.

*Add ½ teaspoon cinnamon and the vanilla.

*Mix to combine.

*Add egg and beat for 1 minute.

*Sift together flours, xanthan gum, baking powder and baking soda and add to cookie mixture.

*Fold in cinnamon chips.

*Roll dough into balls and refrigerate for 15 – 20 minutes.

*Combine remaining ¼ cup sugar and 1½ teaspoon cinnamon in a bowl.

*Roll dough balls in sugar and cinnamon mixture. Coat well.

*Bake on a non-stick sheet pan at 350 degrees about 8 minutes, less if you prefer chewier cookies, more if you prefer crispy cookies.

Flourless Peanut Butter And Chocolate Chip Cookies
by Pam Gordon

Pam has also contributed an apple pie recipe which can be found earlier in this chapter.

This recipe is very easy and good, and it requires no special ingredients. It's good to give to family members who want to prepare something gluten-free. I usually double this recipe because it doesn't make very many.

Flourless Peanut Butter And Chocolate Chip Cookies

Ingredients:
- 1 cup super chunky peanut butter
- 1 cup packed brown sugar
- 1 egg
- 1 teaspoon gluten-free baking soda
- ½ teaspoon gluten-free vanilla
- 1 cup mini semi-sweet chocolate chips

Directions:
    *Preheat oven to 350 degrees.
    *Mix peanut butter, brown sugar, egg, baking soda and vanilla in a medium bowl.
    *Mix in the chocolate chips.
    *Drop dough onto greased cookie sheet (a generous tablespoon) and arrange 2 inches apart.
    *Bake until puffed, golden on bottom and still soft in center.
    *Cool on a cookie sheet for 5 minutes and then transfer to a wire rack to cool completely.

Lemon Curd

by Jessica Duvall

Jessica has also written "Surviving College," which can be read in Chapter Nine, and gives tips for "Planning A Vacation," in Chapter Ten, and "Keeping A Food Diary," in Chapter Twelve.

I use this recipe to top the lemon bundt cake from the Gluten-Free Pantry Cake And Cookie Mix Recipe Book. It also makes a great ice cream topping. It can also be used to make ice cream. It is very easy to make and very YUMMY!! ✍

Lemon Curd

Ingredients:
    3 lemons - zest and juice
    8 ounces caster (fine) sugar
    4 ounces butter
    3 egg yolks - beaten

Directions:
   *Put all the ingredients in the top of a double broiler or in a bowl standing over a pan of simmering water.
   *Heat gently, stirring for about 20 minutes or until the sugar has dissolved and the mixture is thick enough to coat the back of a spoon.
   *Strain the pot, and cover the curd.
   *Store in a cool place and use within 1 month.

Enjoy!

Tips, Tricks And Smiles

Some Simple Celiac Solutions

Don't let celiac disease get you down,
You can find lots of help around town.
Know you're not alone,
Think of this little poem
Join a group, and you won't have to frown.

How To Get Your Doctor's Attention
by Marge Johannemann

Marge has written "Gluten Paranoia," which can be found in Chapter Four and gives some "Cookie Making Tips," later in this chapter.

In these days of HMOs, PPOs, managed care, and increasingly larger physician practices, not to mention voice mail, we all find it harder to be heard as consumers of health care. Here are a few guidelines to help you get the attention you deserve:

1. Select a physician who is knowledgeable about his or her specialty, and is willing to take the time to really listen to what you have to say.

2. Don't waste your physician's time with frivolous conversation and vague information. Make a list of questions in advance to ensure you get all the information you need.

3. For at least two weeks keep a detailed diary of symptoms, diet, episodes or pain, etc., to take to your next appointment. The doctor should find it hard to ignore detailed written information including dates and times.

4. When calling the physician leave a concise message, including time and date of call, your telephone number, and your pharmacy phone number (if necessary). Indicate if your call is an emergency. Allow a reasonable amount of time for the doctor to respond.

5. If your doctor fails to respond, contact the office operator and, in a friendly but firm manner, explain the problem and request a call back by the physician. Always get the name of the person you spoke with.

6. If your doctor still fails to respond, maybe you need to find another physician who is willing to treat you as a health care consumer (his or her "bread and butter").

7. Always remember: You deserve to be treated with respect and dignity. A diagnosis is not a privilege, it is a right.

A Man Named Joe

by Mary Guerriero

My name is Mary Guerriero. I am 61, a legal secretary, and single. I was diagnosed with celiac disease when I was 49. It was the best thing that ever happened to me. I feel great. I'm a little overweight, but am working on that. I have three wonderful adult children and two grandchildren. I spend my spare time working for our support group, the Tri-County Celiac Support Group here in Southeast Michigan, I have been vice-president, president for four years, and am now the secretary.

I find I talk to a lot of people who think it is okay to eat gluten occasionally. I can't stress enough how dangerous this is. It brings to mind a story I heard and would like to share.

There was a man named Joe who lived a good life, believed in God, and regularly attended church services. One day floods were predicted for the area where he lived. The police came and told him he had to leave. Joe refused to go saying, "God will save me." The rains got heavier. A boat came around and told

Joe he had to leave. Joe refused, giving the same reply. A few hours later, with the house nearly covered with water and Joe on the roof, a helicopter came to rescue him. Again, Joe refused to leave, insisting that God would save him. Well, Joe drowned. He got to Heaven, and proceeded to yell at God, saying, "Why didn't you save me?" God replied, "But Joe, I tried to save you. I sent the police, then a boat, and then a helicopter."

I think there is a lesson in this story for all of us. God has sent us our support groups, our gluten-free food companies, and our health food stores. Please don't be tempted to eat gluten. If you are, remember this story. Use your shopping guide. Call other people in your support group if you feel tempted. We care. ✍

I Can't Believe They Said That

by Melonie Katz

Melonie has also written the introduction to the book "What Is Celiac?" and "A Gluten-Free Baker's Dozen And Then Some...," which can be found in Chapter Five.

People's lack of knowledge about celiac disease leads them to say some strange things. How about, "Did you bring your EpiPen to the playgroup in case she eats some wheat?" Yeah, that EpiPen is a multi-purpose tool, huh?

Someone else said, "I had that too and then I outgrew it."

I actually had some woman say to me (when our toddler's belly was so distended, she could have been a poster child for malnourished children): "Wow, she's proud of that big belly, isn't she?"

And my favorite...it's not really so stupid, but it sounds great: "Can she take a gluten pill and then eat gluten?" (Wishful thinking, right?)

Flexible Spending Accounts And Celiac Disease

by Dwight Senne

For at least the last 15 years, I have gone to several doctors with a host of various gastrointestinal disorders. The most common diagnosis I received was irritable bowel syndrome. Finally, in May of 2003, I found a doctor who was thorough enough to check for celiac disease. I have been on the gluten-free diet ever since and feel wonderful!

When first diagnosed with celiac disease, I suppose I was like most people: overwhelmed by the magnitude of the lifestyle change associated with the gluten-free diet. Once reality set in and I began to accept and deal with this new diet, I experienced another overwhelming feeling - the cost of gluten-free foods! While I was not on a tight budget, the idea of spending four times as much for a loaf of bread that was only half the size was daunting to say the least. I immediately began searching for ways to diminish this extra expense.

My research took me to the Internet, where I discovered that according to several IRS rulings (Revenue Ruling 55-

261; Revenue Ruling 76-80, 67 TC 481; Cohen 38 TC 37; Van Kalb TC MEMO 1978 366; Flemming TC MEMO 1980 583) the cost difference between gluten containing food products and specialty gluten-free alternatives is tax deductible for celiac patients. However, it didn't turn out to be that simple.

Further research revealed only that portion which exceeds a 7.5% threshold of adjusted gross income for all medical expenses combined would be deductible. In English, that meant if I had an income of $50,000, I would only be able to deduct my extra expense of gluten-free foods (and any other legally deductible medical expense) that exceeded $3,750 (7.5% of $50,000)! Well, gluten-free foods are not that expensive!

Knowing I would never reach that deductibility threshold, my search continued. Suddenly, a rare epiphany befell me. Since the Internal Revenue Service had ruled specialty foods that are medically necessary to treat a condition are deductible, it may follow that these same expenses may be reimbursable through my employer's Flexible Spending Account program.

Basically, the Flexible Spending Account is a plan that allows you, the employee, to setup a separate savings account, usually administered by a third party. You decide at the beginning of the year how much to contribute to this account. The contributions are deducted from your payroll before tax (meaning you are not charged income tax on the portion of your income you put into the account). As you have out of pocket medical expenses, you file a claim from the Flexible Spending Account administrator for reimbursement of those expenses. Once the account is emptied, no further reimbursements are possible for that year. One caveat with these plans is they are "use it or lose it." This means if you do not have sufficient medical expenses equal to the amount you contributed; you will forfeit any unclaimed balance. Your human resources department should be able to tell you if your company offers a Flexible Spending Account.

In my case, I first called the human resources department at my place of employment to find out if indeed my rationale was valid. The response was, "I don't know, but I doubt it!" Never one to take "no" for an answer (especially when preceded by "I don't know"), I pressed on. A phone call to the Flexible Spending Account administration company yielded the answer I had hoped for: YES!

Fortunately, I happened to connect with a customer service representative who was extremely thorough and diligent. She had to put me on hold several times, but she finally found not only the answer I was looking for but also the proper procedure for filing a claim. She sent out a worksheet I now use to file any claim for gluten-free foods. The sheet has a place to list the food item, cost of the gluten-free variety, cost of the gluten-containing variety, and the price difference. I made several copies of the worksheet, so now whenever I file a claim; I just fill out a new sheet.

The receipts for the food items I am requesting reimbursement for must be included each time with the worksheet. With my first claim, I also had to provide a letter from my doctor clearly stating I was diagnosed with celiac disease and that I must be on a gluten-free diet. They keep this letter on file, so I do not have to send it each time.

Generally speaking, any medical expense the Internal Revenue Service considers deductible (on Schedule A of your

1040 form) is reimbursable. However, employers are not obligated to follow those guidelines. They are not able to add other expenses that are not deductible, but they can delete certain ones (like gluten-free foods) if they choose. So it behooves you to check with your Flexible Spending Account administrator to find out what your plan covers and the proper procedure for reimbursement. It may be necessary to ask to speak to a supervisor, since not every customer service representative will be as helpful as the one I had. You may wish to cite the Internal Revenue Service rulings I listed above to convince them to accept this as a reimbursable item. This can also be helpful in convincing them to reimburse gluten-free food items if they do not currently do so.

While it is still your money that is paying for the entire cost of gluten-free food, using the Flexible Spending Account to switch that money to the tax free variety can add up to significant savings. Depending on the amount of gluten-free food you are buying, and your tax bracket, it can easily be over $100 per year in less taxes you will pay! ✐

Celiac Disease 101

by Donna Griffin

*Donna has also written "Doing Disney World Gluten-Free,"
which can be read in Chapter Ten.*

The time span between our daughter, Jennifer's, diagnosis of celiac disease at "sweet" sixteen and her departure for college seemed to have happened in a flash. Letting go is never easy, letting our now gluten-free daughter loose on a gluten full campus was really not easy.

Initially, we began the college search looking at campuses that had on-campus apartments, with the thought that Jennifer would have access to a (safe) kitchen. Eventually a sensitive, perceptive assistant dean at the university Jennifer now attends, encouraged us to provide Jennifer with a "normal" freshmen experience. This included eating in a campus dining hall with her friends. The challenge would be how to make this idea become a reality.

Having developed a 504 Plan at the high school level, we knew what was ahead of us. First, we asked Jennifer's doctor to update a letter he had written earlier. This stated she had celiac disease, a medical condition that required a medically restricted diet. Then, in developing the 504 Plan itself, we outlined those reasonable accommodations that would be necessary to give Jen equal access to the college campus. Essentially these included:

1. Access to a refrigerator and freezer for the storage of perishable gluten-free food.

2. Access to a separate microwave and toaster oven in order to prepare gluten-free food and to avoid cross-contamination of these items.

3. Participation in a dining plan that would offer her gluten-free meals.

4. Access to storage space for non-perishable gluten-free food items.

Next, we met with the food services supervisor, early in August, before the start of classes. At that meeting we discussed specific points; for example, where exactly would her perishable and non-perishable items be stored and where her "utensils" (colander, toaster, etc.) would safely be kept. Finally we agreed upon how to obtain her gluten-free food.

As luck would have it, "gluten-free angels" placed a health food store in the middle of rural, central Pennsylvania, stocked with celiac friendly food! The dining services personnel even arranged to shop there on a regular basis because Jennifer was not permitted to have a car on campus. At that initial meeting Jennifer was introduced to the dining staff, so they would recognize the young lady who would be going into otherwise forbidden territory in the kitchen.

Moving in day we arrived with colander in hand. They had "dedicated" a toaster, freezer/refrigerator, shelves and a storage cabinet for Jennifer. She and the dining staff were in business!

Once classes started, the dining staff made arrangements for certain meals to be prepared ahead of time, so when Jennifer arrived (especially for dinner), she wouldn't have to wait to eat. The other connection we made was with the Office of Residential Life. They agreed to waive certain restrictions regarding the ability to keep a toaster oven in her dorm room. In addition, she was given a room with a little more storage space, so she had a place to keep her gluten-free munchies. By her junior year she was given priority in being assigned an on campus "condo" with a kitchenette. By this time her roommates were more than familiar with how to safely share a kitchen with Jennifer and she was well on her way to independent gluten-free living.

Speaking about those gluten-free angels, Jennifer pledged a sorority in her sophomore year. Guess what? Unbeknownst to Jennifer, her sponsor, also known as her pledge "mom," was a celiac too!

Since Jennifer's freshman year, I have received many phone calls from anxious parents planning life for their college bound celiac young adults. I have noticed each year more and more speak about how receptive many campuses have been. Although I find this encouraging, my best advice still is, don't rely on a well-meaning college admissions officer. Get yourself and your college bound celiac into the kitchen! 🖊

Donna's daughter, Jennifer, has written "When You're A Teen," which can be read in Chapter Seven.

Cookie Making Tips

by Marge Johannemann

Marge has also written the pieces "Gluten Paranoia," which can be read in Chapter Four, and "How To Get Your Doctor's Attention," which can be read earlier in this chapter.

I have put together these tips after a lot of trial and error and experimenting over the years. I hope they're helpful.

1. Real butter makes the best cookies. I recommend unsalted butter.

2. Use brown rice flour or bean flour instead of white rice flour to provide extra fiber.

3. Omit potato starch and tapioca starch for a firmer, less fragile cookie.

4. Xanthan gum is not needed for cookies.

5. Natural sweeteners, such as raw sugar, beet sugar, or brown sugar, can be used in place of refined sugar for a healthier alternative. Natural sweeteners are metabolized faster and put less of a load on the pancreas, which is especially important for diabetics.

6. Replace ½ to 1 cup of rice or bean flour with soy flour for a chewy cookie.

7. Don't be afraid to experiment or adapt wheat recipes into a gluten-free form. It's fun and provides variety. ✍

Keep A Food Diary

by Jessica Duvall

Jessica has also written the piece "Surviving College," which can be read in Chapter Nine, tips for "Planning A Vacation," which can be read in Chapter Ten, and a recipe for "Lemon Curd," which can be found in Chapter Eleven.

Here is a thought for those of you who have just been diagnosed. It worked for me. In the beginning it is a good idea to keep a food diary. Write down everything that goes into your mouth, how much you ate, and what time you ate it. Then, if and when you have a reaction, you can trace it back to the problem.

When starting the diet I would stick to very plain meat, veggies, and potatoes. Even the smallest spice, dairy, or extra grease can make your tummy hurt. Your body is trying to heal and adding extra "stuff" can make it difficult.

You need to learn how to pay attention to your body. If you notice extra hair loss, bloating, pains, etc., you might have ingested gluten. Your body is a pretty amazing thing and it lets you know when it's not happy and healthy. Your tummy is very sensitive right now. Keep it simple, pay attention and it will be easier. ✍

Beware:
Hidden Contamination
by Valerie Bernes

Valerie has also written "An Unusual Discovery," which can be read in Chapter One.

Even though certain products may not list any gluten-containing ingredients, there still may be traces of gluten in the product. Let's take for example, corn chips. One company lists their ingredients as corn, oil, and salt; sounds safe. Beware! I called the company and found out they process all of their products (gluten-free and gluten containing) on the same equipment. Even if they clean the equipment between runs (as they say they do) they must not clean it well enough for sensitive celiacs, like me. I get reactions from all of their products whether gluten is listed in the ingredients or not. The same is true for other products that "should" be safe: such as local grocery store rice, or certain brands of corn meal.

I must say from the time I discovered I had celiac disease (1997) until early 2003, I was able to tolerate small amounts of gluten in my diet, but not anymore. Contaminated products pose a problem for celiacs who must remain 100% gluten-free. Recently, some local groceries have begun injecting their chickens with solutions to keep them moist. While I haven't written to complain, I've had reactions to this "minimally processed" chicken, so I assume there's something in the solution that contains gluten. Another roadblock to deal with.

There is a website with a list of contaminated products. Check it out:

http://geocities.com/HotSprings/Spa/4003/gf-contaminated.html ✍

Spread The Kindness
by Jessica Duvall

Jessica has also written "Surviving College," which can be read in Chapter Nine, has contributed a recipe "Lemon Curd," which can be read in Chapter Eleven, and has given tips on "Planning A Vacation," in Chapter Ten and on "Keeping A Food Diary," earlier in this chapter.

I am very much a believer in giving back when you have received something great. It has only been a short time since my diagnosis and many people have been very kind to me along the way. They have not asked for a "thank you," instead they have simply asked for me to pass on good things to others in return for the good things I received. Here is a great moment when I have given something back, but also gotten something in return.

My happiest gluten-free moment recently has been making sure a boy on my brother's football team has a gluten-free lunch to take on the team bus for all the away games and a gluten-free dinner for after the home games just as the other players do. This child has gone without and has been excluded for a while now. Once I found out he had celiac disease I made it a very high priority to make sure he had his own sack lunch. I make sure when the other boys have a brownie, he has a gluten-free treat in his sack. For away games he gets rollups and the boys get sandwiches. He LOVES it!!

The best part was, after he got his first meal from our family, he came up and gave me a huge hug and told me "thank you." What a wonderful gift to me for a 16-year-old boy to give an adult a hug. That was all I needed to know. He was no longer feeling left out!!

Spread the kindness. Not only will you help someone else but you'll feel great too. 🖊

Keys To Gluten-Free Kids

by Lindsay Amadeo

Lindsay has also contributed recipes for "Gluten-Free Play Materials," and a "Sample Letter To School Teachers," both of which can be found in Chapter Six.

My son, Sam, was the first person in our family to be diagnosed with celiac disease. He was 15 months old and had gone from a fat and happy one-year-old, to a child I began to fear was going to die three months later. I will never forget that feeling of terror when I started to believe I might lose my child if someone couldn't find out what was wrong with him. The thing I dreaded most was telling his three-year-old brother that "his" baby was sick. I am ever grateful for the very manageable outcome of celiac disease.

Five years later and happily gluten-free, here are my best tips for children at different ages:

For all ages:
*   Decide what your gluten-free philosophy is at each age and stage.

*   Are you going to have a gluten-free household or a co-mingled gluten/gluten-free home?

*   Will you go to great lengths to make sure your child doesn't feel different, or will you teach him to accept his differences?

*   Are you going to only choose products produced on dedicated gluten-free lines for fear of cross-contamination or will you use gluten-free "mainstream" products?

*   Knowing where you stand on the spectrum will relieve you of much agony. And you can always change your stance to best fit your circumstances over time.

*   Get some of the well recognized gluten-free product lists, such as the one from the Celiac Sprue Association (www.csausa.org).

*   Call ahead. Always. Call restaurants, check for health food stores before you travel, etc.

*   When traveling, get hotel rooms with a kitchenette. And a pool, of course!

*   Kids are very matter of fact. Present the disease and the diet in a straightforward manner: "you have blue eyes and cannot eat gluten, but you can...."

For toddlers:

Keep it simple with toddlers. A key developmental goal is for them to begin to understand that certain types of food "hurt your tummy" or whatever the bothersome symptom is.

Ideas to manage the diet at this age:

* Keep a supply of a favorite treat in the diaper bag. Sam would choose M&Ms over anything and these often came in handy when he spotted a gluten treat he could not have.

* This one may seem silly but if you are going to a large party, picnic, or potluck consider putting a "do not feed me" sticker on your child. We have a large extended family of older women that would not think twice about giving the toddler a cracker. A reminder was very helpful.

* Although you might think this is disgusting, they are toddlers, so be careful of the dog's dish and make sure to pick up food off of the floor.

* Be patient with toilet training, as loose stools can make getting the job done a little tricky.

For preschoolers:

Establish a warm connection with your child's teacher and emphasize the need for good communication when food is involved. This is very important in these years.

Ideas to manage the diet at this age:

* Send the teacher, principal and other caregivers a letter a few weeks before school starts. I have found teachers are quickly confused when I try to explain the disease and diet. I have had much more luck focusing on communication as the important issue. Most teachers are familiar with food allergies and quickly grasp the most important aspects. (I've submitted a sample letter which I use that can be found in Chapter Six of this book.)

* Ask for a list of classmate birthdays and holiday parties so you can pre-plan.

* Put a plastic tub of snacks and other goodies together for the teacher to keep in the classroom.

* Freeze cupcakes ahead of time so you can easily defrost one. Ice it and send it to school on class birthdays.

*Consider a medic-alert bracelet in these years. Even

if the teacher remembers, parent volunteers will often set a gluten treat down in front of your child and the bracelet is a good reminder.

* Consider providing gluten-free play dough, pasta, etc., for the entire class. If that is not possible, find out what type of play materials you need to provide for your child. (I have submitted recipes for gluten-free play materials which can be found in Chapter 6.)

* A homeroom parent very often gets an early notice of upcoming food related events. Either become the homeroom parent or if that's not possible develop a line of communication with her.

Most children accept differences in their friends. However, their natural curiosity often leads to questions. Consider reading one of the children's celiac storybooks or provide this demonstration: Cut a looped terry cloth towel into strips. Give each child one to handle and talk about how the bumpy side has loops to grab vitamins from food and carry them into the body. Then, talk about how the smooth side doesn't have any bumps to grab the vitamins and that this is what happens when someone with celiac disease eats gluten.

Point out to your child that everyone has differences. Explain that some kids are allergic to dogs; some cannot eat peanuts, etc.

For grade school:

This is the age where the parent must begin transferring responsibility for the diet to the child. This can be very hard when you have taken such active charge for so long. But the diet belongs to the child and they must learn to manage on their own eventually. All of the preschool tips apply as well as:

* Call the birthday party host parent ahead of time and let them know your child has a food intolerance and must bring his own cupcake. Ask about other foods they will be serving. Very often the ice cream, juice, etc. can be gluten-free if the host is open to your suggesting a brand. Remember the emphasis is on the birthday child and the good time all the kids will be having that is unrelated to food.

* Call a sleepover host parents as well. Find out what is for dinner, breakfast, and snack. Pack gluten-free cold cereal, popcorn, and other treats in your child's overnight bag.

* Most sports teams have a snack after the game. Bring a gluten-free choice for your child and sign up several times to take your turn for gluten-free snacks all around.

* Public schools are required to provide a gluten-free hot lunch for your child.

However, their ability to do so without contamination depends on the particular staff. You have to decide what you are comfortable with. Meet with the district dietician and determine what is practical.

*   Transfer responsibility. Don't assume you know how the child wants to handle each social situation. Ask each time. Some days my children want a decorated cupcake for the birthday party, other times they eat from their school box. Occasionally they will decide to eat ahead of time and just concentrate on the fun.

*   Make sure you teach your kids to cook. They will have to do so for themselves. Even more so than other people.

*   Teach your child to order for themselves in restaurants.

And that is as far as I can go. Right now my celiac kids are in first and third grades. Middle school, high school, college and beyond are still ahead of us.

Here's to a wonderful gluten-free future.

Social Celiac Course 101
by Leslie Elsner

*Leslie has also written "Don't Keep Celiac Disease A Secret,"
which can be read in Chapter Nine and "Top Ten New Year's
Resolutions," which can be read later in this chapter.*

Arm yourself with these coping techniques when you
attend a party:

Chapter 1 — Cocktails

When the bartender asks, "What's your
poison?" this may not be so far off. Most hard
liquors are likely made from one of the various
grains celiacs must avoid. There are a few
relatively safe options: most wine, tequila, and
rum. Or you can always opt for gluten-free
soda or juice; no one will be the wiser when
you join in on the traditional party toast.

Chapter 2 — Hors D'oeuvres

These little critters will most likely be off
your list. Most are wrapped in some sort of
dough [or sauce] that is not likely to be gluten-

free. Fresh fruit or veggies may be your best hope. Better yet, keep a small bag of gluten-free goodies with you to eat while everyone else stuffs themselves with pigs in a blanket.

Chapter 3 – Entrees

This gets a little more difficult, but don't despair. If you are celebrating in a restaurant, try to speak to the chef or maitre d' and advise them of your situation. If possible, try to reach them prior to the meal. Remember to stay away from anything with stuffing, dressings with unknown ingredients, or fried foods cooked in the same oil as breaded foods. When dining at someone's home, offer to bring a homemade dish to contribute to the meal. Your host will be thankful for the help, and you will be sure to have at least one gluten-free option when you eat.

Chapter 4 – Dessert

This is the time you may start to feel a little sorry for yourself. That is, until you see the stuffed look on your dining companions' faces. While you may opt for fresh fruit or a light gluten-free Sorbet, they can barely speak or move because they are so full from that rich chocolate cake. So give yourself a pat on the back and remember, it's just one less hour on the treadmill for you at the gym.

Tips From Mary Guerriero
by Mary Guerriero

Mary has also written "A Man Named Joe," which can be read earlier in this chapter.

*   Try to strike a good balance between being totally paranoid about gluten and taking it too lightly. You shouldn't be afraid to leave your own kitchen, but we also don't go out for pizza and beer with the guys.

*   Use your restaurant card when you go out to eat. It helps to validate your need for special attention and it helps the chef know what is and is not safe for you.

*   Remember ingredients can change anytime. The barbecue sauce that was gluten-free the last time you bought it might not be gluten-free the next time. Constantly update and check with manufacturers.

* If you live with non-celiacs, then make sure you mark all the gluten-free items with stickers. If possible, have one shelf in the pantry for gluten-free products, and make sure the others in your home know not to touch anything on that shelf. (Why, you ask? Gluten-free items are costly; once they are gone you can't usually go to the local store and easily replace them; and finally, a non-celiac could contaminate your food items with bread crumbs, etc.)

* Unless everyone in the house eats gluten-free bread, you need to have a separate toaster that no one else uses, or use a toaster oven you can wipe out before you use it.

* Use separate condiments or make sure the non-celiacs you live with know not to contaminate the condiments by dipping knives, spoons, etc. back in after touching regular bread. Yes, those few crumbs really do matter, even if you don't get immediate symptoms, you are still damaging your gut.

* Don't lick envelopes and stamps; the glue may come from a gluten source.

* When you are first diagnosed, shop the perimeter of your grocery store. Fresh fruits, vegetables, and meats are going to be

safe and you will not be prepared to read and understand labels for awhile.

*   As a newly diagnosed celiac I suggest if an item has more than five ingredients, or ingredients you can't pronounce, then don't buy it. Later, after you begin to understand the diet better, you can start adding other ingredients that are safe.

*   Don't assume every time something goes wrong it is because of gluten or celiac disease. Celiacs are just as likely as non-celiacs to have other problems. Both celiacs and non-celiacs can sometimes have stomach aches due to viruses, spoiled food, other allergies/sensitivities, etc.

*   Ask your favorite health food store to carry gluten-free products.

*   The best place to buy rice flour is at an Indian store; you pay $2.49 or less for 5 pounds. You might also check Asian stores for items such as potato starch and tapioca starch.

*   At McDonald's, Wendy's, and Burger King, the french fries should be safe so long as they are cooked in their own oil, separate from all other fried foods. Most fast food

restaurants do cook the fries separately, so the taste isn't affected by other fried foods. Just be sure to ask at your local fast food restaurants.

* If you have e-mail, there is a free e-mail list for celiacs. To subscribe, send a message to:

listserv@maelstrom.stjohns.edu
containing this line:
SUBSCRIBE CELIAC Firstname Lastname

* At the time of this writing, Wendy's baked potatoes, with all the toppings, are gluten-free. Their chili, taco salad (including sour cream), and taco chips are also gluten-free. The GRILLED chicken breast is also gluten-free, without the sauce; but don't confuse this with the breaded chicken breast which is not gluten-free. Frosties are also gluten-free.

* Don't let celiac disease define who you are. You are a unique person with many traits and facets to your life, who just happens to have celiac disease. In a perfect world there would be no diseases, but as diseases go, celiac is real doable. The longer you are on the diet the more you will realize you can substitute for just about anything that normally has gluten in it.

Top Ten New Year's Resolutions

by Leslie Elsner

Leslie has also written "Don't Keep Celiac Disease A Secret," which can be read in Chapter Nine and "Social Celiac Course 101," which can be read earlier in this chapter.

1. **Check food items BEFORE you put them in your mouth:**
   If there is any doubt as to the safety of the ingredients, skip them. It's better to be safe than sorry. Continuously check back with manufacturers as they may change ingredients and suppliers.

2. **Join your local support group:**
   Not only is it a great place to meet new friends, trade tips and recipes, but where else can you find more empathetic listeners and be able to share gluten-free goodies?

3. **Volunteer to help those newly diagnosed:**
   Remember the confusion and helplessness you felt at the beginning and channel that into helping others gain from your knowledge and experience.

4. **Broaden your culinary horizons:**
   Try trading recipes and helpful tips with fellow celiacs. Start with something simple. If you are new to the kitchen you will soon find what a little experimenting can do.

5. **Have an annual checkup:**
   Even if you feel terrific, it is important to have a yearly checkup that includes testing of serum antibodies, vitamin levels, and annual blood workups. Once you have attained good health, keep yourself there.

6. **Exercise regularly:**
   A healthy body is not only attained by good eating habits. Diet and exercise together can help to strengthen your bones, relieve stress and improve your mental state.

7. **Don't minimize your condition:**
   It should be taken quite seriously and others will take their cue from how you present it. The serious implications of not following a strict gluten-free diet must never be taken lightly.

8. **Encourage family members to be tested:**
   Since many family members may be asymptomatic, this testing is crucial in protecting your loved ones from serious consequences.

9. **Get the word out:**
   There's no reason to keep celiac disease a secret. Share your knowledge and expertise with your physicians and health care providers. Even those who are knowledgeable on celiac disease can always learn a helpful tip or two which you have experienced first hand.

10. **Keep a positive outlook:**
    Remember how far you have come and how much better you feel. Give yourself a pat on the back for making a choice for a healthy life.

Take A Deep Slow Breath
by Pat Bridges

I was diagnosed at the age of 57, after decades of increasingly uncomfortable, miserable symptoms. After my diagnosis, life was brand new! Painful osteoarthritis gradually became more bearable, migraines disappeared, and even my personality changed for the better.

When my children left home, I began volunteering at schools and the local hospital. Now, I restrict myself to hospital volunteer work, which I've been enjoying for over 15 years. Apart from the constant effort to keep my weight down, I'm healthy and happy.

If you've just been diagnosed here are a few tips for you. I hope they help.

*Take a deep, slow breath. Make this the first confident breath you take when you embark on your gluten-free life.

*There is no cure, but there is no need for prescribed medication.

*There is no cure, but you know recovery is possible.

*There is no cure, but you know that you alone are in charge of that recovery.

How much better can it get?

Your recovery will be amazing. Complete recovery time differs from person to person. For me it was many months, but I knew within a couple of weeks that gluten-free was for me.

Since then, years of misery have become a dim memory and life will never be the same again. Remember that life throws us a curve from time to time. In our case, a very small minority of us may not be completely curable. If that happens, take that deep, slow breath and face the new challenge with the same confidence that only you can manage.

You have all of us for support. Use it and embrace it. Good luck!

Give Us Your Personal Touch

A Personal Touch Publishing invites you to send us your comments and thoughts about this book and to suggest topics for future books in this series. You can do this by visiting our Web site at www.apersonaltouchon.com.

When you're at our Web site you can find our other helpful titles and the new ones we're working on. We are also accepting submissions for "A Personal Touch On...™ Celiac Disease, part II. So, if you feel you have something more to contribute send us your story, recipes, tips, etc. and help others with celiac disease.

Become part of the Personal Touch family by submitting a piece and sharing your experiences to help others. It's easy and not only will others benefit, but you'll feel great too, knowing that you helped someone.

To order copies of
"A Personal Touch On...™"
Books ✍
visit our website at:
www.apersonaltouchon.com